Chronic Pain
A Primer for Physicians

D1550292

The authors and publisher have undertaken reasonable steps to ensure that the information contained in this publication is correct at the time of printing. These steps have included checking the information against generally accepted sources and submitting the publication to peer review.

Despite these steps, the authors and publisher cannot guarantee that the information is or will remain correct and complete. The sources which they have used and the peer review process are by no means infallible. Developments in medical and/or clinical knowledge may show, or suggest, that some or all of the information is incorrect, incomplete or misleading.

Accordingly, neither the authors nor the publisher nor any other person involved in the production of this publication can accept any legal responsibility for any loss or damage caused by the use of any of the information contained in this publication, except when that loss and damage has been caused by their own negligence.

Since there is a possibility that the information contained in this publication may be incorrect, incomplete or misleading, and the consequences of acting upon information which is incorrect, incomplete or misleading could be very serious, readers are strongly advised to take steps to verify the information contained in this publication prior to using it. Before using information relating to any drug or piece of medical equipment, particularly those which are new and/or unfamiliar, it is essential that readers consult the most recent version of the drug or equipment manufacturer's product literature to verify that the information is both accurate and up-to-date.

Published by Remedica
1 New Oxford Street, London, WC1A 1NU, UK
20 N Wacker Drive, Suite 1642, Chicago, IL 60606, USA
Tel: +44 (0)20 7759 2999
Fax: +44 (0)20 7759 2951
E-mail: info@remedicabooks.com
www.remedicabooks.com

Publisher: Andrew Ward
Commissioning Editor: Charlotte Palmer
Editor: Catherine Booth
Production Manager: Mary Hughes
Design and Artwork: AS&K Skylight

1-905721-46-3
978-1-905721-46-7

Printed in Canada

Chronic Pain
A Primer for Physicians

MARCO PAPPAGALLO, MD
Director, Pain Medicine Research and Development
Professor, Department of Anesthesiology
Mount Sinai School of Medicine
New York, USA

MADS WERNER, MD, PhD
Associate Professor
Department of Oncology
Lund University Hospital
Sweden

With contribution from:
MORRIS FRASER
De Zwarte Hond
Noordhoekstraat 50
De Panne
Belgium

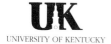

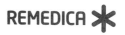

Jointly sponsored by the University of Kentucky and Remedica Medical Education and Publishing. Supported by an unrestricted educational grant from Cephalon.

CME information

Disclosures

Mads Werner, MD, PhD, and Morris Fraser have no relevant financial relationships to disclose. Marco Pappagallo, MD has relationships with Anesiva, Elan, Endo Pharmaceuticals, GlaxoSmithKline, Merck & Co., Inc., the National Institutes of Health, and Roche Pharmaceuticals.

Accreditation

This activity has been planned and implemented in accordance with the Essential Areas and policies of the Accreditation Council for Continuing Medical Education through the joint sponsorship of the University of Kentucky College of Medicine and Remedica Medical Education and Publishing. The University of Kentucky College of Medicine is accredited by the ACCME to provide continuing medical education for physicians.

The University of Kentucky College of Medicine designates this educational activity for a maximum of eight (8.0) *AMA PRA Category 1 Credits*™. Physicians should only claim credit commensurate with the extent of their participation in the activity.

The University of Kentucky College of Medicine presents this activity for educational purposes only. Participants are expected to utilize their own expertise and judgment while engaged in the practice of medicine. The content of the presentations is provided solely by presenters who have been selected for presentations because of recognized expertise in their field.

Instructions for obtaining CME credit

Participation in this activity should be completed in approximately 8 hours. A passing score of 70% or higher is required for issue of a statement of credit. To successfully complete this program and receive credit, participants must follow these steps:

1. Read the learning objectives (below).
2. Read the book's text and tables, and review the figures.
3. Read, complete, and submit answers to the self-assessment questions at the back of the book. Participants must respond to all self-assessment and program evaluation questions to receive a certificate by mail.
4. Complete the registration form.
5. Visit the University of Kentucky's website at www.cecentral.com/getcredit/, enter the program code MEN07150, and follow the online instructions. Alternatively, return the post-test answer sheet, program evaluation form, and registration form (or a photocopy of all) to the address provided.

Needs statement

Chronic pain presents a significant burden to society in terms of lost workforce productivity and significant healthcare resource utilization and cost. Indeed, chronic pain is one of the most common reasons that patients consult a physician. Yet, despite the existence of safe and effective therapies (including antidepressants, anticonvulsants, and opioids), pain is commonly undertreated. The most common obstacles to effective pain management are patient underreporting, inadequate assessment, lack of knowledge about available treatments, and inadequate treatment. *Chronic Pain: A Primer for Physicians*, a CME-accredited educational program, is designed to provide physicians with an overview of the current state-of-the-art in relation to the diagnosis and management of chronic pain and thereby lead to improvements in patient outcomes.

Learning objectives
Goal

The goal of this activity is to assist healthcare providers in the management of patients with chronic pain.

Objectives

Upon completion of this activity, the reader should be able to:

- Understand the different presentations of chronic pain.
- Appreciate the main classes of therapeutics available for the management of a range of chronic pain indications.
- Identify effective clinical strategies for the use of opioids, including rapid-onset opioids, in patients with chronic pain.
- Understand the principles of an effective risk-management strategy for the use of opioids in patients with chronic pain.
- Understand the complementary actions of nonpharmacologic strategies, and when these should be used in patients with chronic pain.

Date of release: 1 December 2007
Date of expiration: 1 December 2008

Foreword

Pain is a leading reason for patients to seek care in virtually all healthcare settings. Traditional medical teaching instructs us that when an individual presents with a pain complaint, the best approach to help is through the creation of a differential diagnosis based upon a logical regression of likely anatomic or physiologic disorders. When a tissue-related etiology cannot be determined, the differential diagnosis turns toward 'nonorganic' or 'psychological' causes. This is how we (the medical profession) have been taught – and continue to be taught, especially in our clinical training years – and so, quite understandably, this is how we act.

But the knowledge about pain, its mechanisms, and modes of treatment has changed, and so it is time to modify our thinking and the behaviors that follow. Pain as a disease state – that is, a distinct neuropathological condition that may persist, independent of any ongoing structural lesion, infection, mechanical trauma, or ischemia – is still too new as an emerging concept (notwithstanding its rapidly deepening scientific underpinnings) to have gained either widespread awareness or acceptance throughout the mainstream healthcare professions. So when will the differential diagnosis of a patient with chronic pain that is not attributable to an evident concurrent somatic or visceral pathologic finding include 'rule out neuropathological pain state' (or 'maldynia' as some have called it)? When will we be able to prevent chronic pain or limit the extraordinary morbidity that it causes by employing new knowledge? When will the 'tipping point' occur?

These rhetorical questions are not immediately answerable, because change theory tells us that the trajectory toward a shift in thinking, which finally yields to an adoption of not-necessarily-brand-new-but-now-timely-and-relevant knowledge (no less translating this into day-to-day practice), can vary considerably. Peer-reviewed technical publications of advances in neuroscience and pharmacology, including breakthroughs that provide entirely new research and diagnostic tools, exemplified by imaging and receptor cloning techniques, are not commonly sought after or immediately accessible to busy physicians. Most physicians simply do not have the time or highly specialized knowledge in these emerging basic science domains to create a practical clinical context for these reports.

A cogent summary, on the other hand, can rapidly and thoroughly update and inspire understanding while providing utility for immediate problem-solving. *Chronic Pain: A Primer for Physicians* is such a medium and catalyst for positive change. It is a comprehensible, readily 'digestible', and applicable handbook that provides an 'ah ha' experience, enticing the reader into a frame shift in thinking about our all-too-common medical nemesis: persistent pain. This 'primer' compiles and condenses a huge body of material. It starts off by grounding both the neophyte and veteran physician alike in the most up-to-date substrates of 'the pain system' and uses this essential foundation to provide a 'soup-to-nuts' tour of what every physician needs to know to help patients with problematic pain. It is time for physicians – and their patients – to experience gratification, rather than frustration, in the face of these challenging conditions. This book will help; let the 'tipping' begin!

Perry G Fine, MD
Professor of Anesthesiology, Pain Research Center,
School of Medicine, University of Utah
Senior Fellow for Medical Leadership, National Hospice
and Palliative Care Organization, Alexandria
Chairman, National Initiative on Pain Control
(see www.painknowledge.com)

Contents

Introduction

According to the International Association for the Study of Pain, an operational definition of chronic pain is pain that has persisted beyond the normal tissue healing time, usually taken to be 3 months.

A large number of patients suffer from chronic pain, but what is the prevalence?

Pain is one of the most common reasons why patients seek medical advice from their physician. The American Pain Society estimates that 50 million Americans are partially or totally disabled by pain. This striking statistic is certain to increase as our population continues to age. In order to combat this growing problem, healthcare professionals must arm themselves with information. By developing the appropriate pain assessment skills, and by staying abreast of the rapidly changing therapies used in pain management, clinicians can play an important role in improving the quality of life of those living with pain.

According to the Joint Commission on the Accreditation of Healthcare Organizations, one-third of Americans will experience chronic pain at some point in their lives. Chronic pain costs the economy billions of dollars in lost productivity every year, and is a major cause of absenteeism from work.

According to a survey conducted by Roper Starch Worldwide Inc. in 1998 and released in January 1999, patients with chronic pain have trouble finding doctors who can treat their pain. Reportedly, on average, one in four patients had changed physicians at least three times due to multiple reasons, including "Pain not taken seriously by the physician," "Doctors' lack of knowledge about chronic pain," and "Inadequate pain management." According to a telephone survey based on 800 interviews with adults experiencing chronic pain and conducted in 2004 by Roper Public Affairs and Media, approximately 75% of individuals with chronic pain have lived in pain for >3 years. Among this group, one-third have lived in pain for >10 years. Of note, a large number of patients with chronic pain have concerns about taking pain medications for the rest of their lives, drug-related side effects, and risk of addiction. Nearly 50% of respondents said that their pain was not under control.

Finally, according to the 2006 National Center for Health Statistics Report, released by the Centers for Disease Control and Prevention's National Center for Health Statistics (www.cdc.gov/nchs/hus.htm), one in four adults reported pain for at least 24 hours during the past month, and one in 10 reported chronic pain. Low back pain, headache, and knee pain were the most common complaints. More than 25% of the adults interviewed said that they had experienced low back pain in the previous 3 months; 15% of adults reported migraine or severe headache in the previous 3 months. Reports of severe joint pain increased with age.

Multiple barriers to appropriate pain management have been identified. These include inadequate medical education, an insufficient number of healthcare professionals trained in the care of patients with chronic pain, and healthcare system difficulty in the recognition of pain relief as a quality of life priority.

In 2006, International Communications Research conducted an internet survey for the American Pain Foundation. Out of 303 chronic pain sufferers on opioid therapy who were included in the final sample, 60% reported breakthrough pain at least once a day, with considerable impact on their quality of life. In addition, more than half of the surveyed patients reported being depressed, difficulty with mental concentration, and inability to sleep at night. Approximately 75% of patients expressed a need for new and better treatment options for their pain; only 14% reported satisfaction with their current medications.

How are different pains classified?

Pain can be classified according to:
- duration (eg, acute, chronic)
- cause (eg, malignancy, ischemia, infection, trauma)
- anatomic region (eg, back pain, neck pain, headache, chest pain)
- temporal characteristics (eg, acute pain, chronic pain, daily pain, intermittent/recurrent pain, constant pain, breakthrough pain)
- organ system (eg, pancreatic pain, plexopathy, musculoskeletal pain, arthritic pain)
- mechanism (eg, nociceptive, inflammatory, neuropathic)
- syndrome (eg, chronic back pain, complex regional pain syndrome, fibromyalgia, chronic daily headache)

Pain taxonomy has traditionally separated pain states into two broad categories: nociceptive and neuropathic.

Nociceptive pain

Nociceptive pain resulting from a tissue injury – either in somatic structures such as the skin, mucosa, muscles, or joints (nociceptive somatic pain) or visceral structures (nociceptive visceral pain) – activates pain receptors (nociceptors), leading to pain perception. The nociceptive signal presumably originates from 'healthy' tissue nociceptors that are activated or sensitized by the local release of allogeneic substances (eg, protons, prostaglandins, bradykinin, adenosine, cytokines). Nociceptive pain is often responsive to analgesics such as acetaminophen (paracetamol), nonsteroidal anti-inflammatory drugs (NSAIDs), and opioids.

Neuropathic pain

In neuropathic pain, the pain signal is generated ectopically and abnormally by peripheral and/or central nervous system (CNS) pain pathways.

Common types of neuropathic pain are painful diabetic neuropathy, postherpetic neuralgia following shingles, phantom pain following amputation, posttraumatic nerve injury, radiculopathy, postamputation stump pain, and complex regional pain syndrome.

What are the optimal strategies in the management of chronic pain?

It is commonly accepted that a prerequisite for the successful management of chronic pain is a multidisciplinary and multiprofessional approach. A simple pathophysiologic model may be used to outline multimodal management strategies.

The mechanisms involved in the passage from an acute pain state to chronic pain are complex, multiple, and still poorly understood. Research in this area is obviously very important. The few clinical studies available have concentrated on the development of chronic pain following:

- various surgical procedures (eg, postmastectomy syndrome, postherniotomy syndrome)
- postherpetic neuralgia following herpes zoster (shingles)
- chronic low back pain following recurrent attacks of acute back pain

Pain is often associated with immobilization either due to movement-related excessive increases in pain or enforced restrictions (eg, bed rest, cast). Both of these can lead to physical deconditioning and disability, which may aggravate and promote the development of chronic pain. Moreover, limb immobilization following a traumatic injury (nociceptive pain) is also known to play a role in the genesis of a neuropathic pain

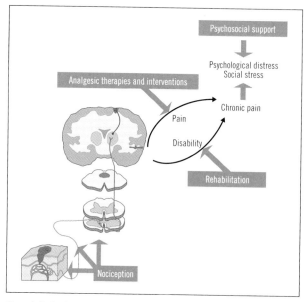

Figure 1. Pathophysiologically based management targets in chronic pain.

condition called complex regional pain syndrome/reflex sympathetic dystrophy (see **Chapter 8**).

Management strategies should firstly include avoidance of chronic pain by the aggressive treatment of acute pain, particularly recurrent pain, with analgesics (acetaminophen, local anesthetics, NSAIDs, and opioids) (see **Figure 1**).

Rehabilitation measures (eg, mobilization, exercise, physical therapy) become possible as a consequence of effective pharmacologic pain therapy. Increased mobilization may help to prevent the development of chronic pain. Psychosocial support and patient education, provided in a professional and empathic manner, are important methods that may augment other treatment modalities and improve the patient's pain-coping strategies.

Marco Pappagallo, MD and Mads Werner, MD, PhD

Reading material

1. Pappagallo M, Editor. *The Neurological Basis of Pain*. New York: McGraw-Hill, 2005.
2. Benzon HT, Raja SN, Molloy RE, et al., Editors. *Essentials of Pain Medicine and Regional Anesthesia*, 2nd edn. London: Churchill Livingstone, 2004.
3. Wallace MS, Staats PS, Editors. *Pain Medicine and Management: Just the Facts*. New York: McGraw-Hill, 2004

1 • Physiology of pain

During the past decades, we have witnessed an increased understanding of the mechanisms that initiate and maintain pain. Effective and rational pain management requires an understanding of the different types of pain and the key processes that operate in each type.

What is pain?

In 1979, the International Association for the Study of Pain published its first working definition of pain: "An unpleasant sensory and emotional experience associated with actual or potential tissue damage, or described in terms of such damage" [1].

This definition was reaffirmed in 1994, but with some amendments. In particular, it was recognized that pain could occur in the absence of tissue damage and that it is impacted by psychological factors [2]. Pain is subjective; therefore, everyone experiences and expresses it differently. Present-day definitions of pain have to take into account factors such as:

- the situation in which the pain occurs
- fear factors (eg, concern about serious illness)
- emotions (eg, depression, optimism)
- existential issues
- cultural factors (eg, emotional dependence, stoicism)

Types of pain

For a pragmatic clinical approach, pain can be divided into two broad categories:

- nociceptive pain
- neuropathic pain

Nociceptive pain

Nociceptive pain is the physiological process that occurs within the body during the activation and sensitization of tissue nociceptors, also known as $A\delta$ and C *nerve fibers*. By definition, nociceptive pain is initiated and maintained through the activity of undamaged (ie, presumably molecularly intact or physiologically 'healthy') nerve fibers. These small nerve fibers can respond to thermal stimuli (eg, heat, cold), mechanical stimuli (eg, pinch, pressure, stretch), and chemical stimuli (eg, low pH) from damaged cells.

Inflammatory products (eg, prostanoids, bradykinin, cytokines) can sensitize nociceptors to a range of mechanical, thermal, and chemical stimuli. Notably, a proportion of the afferent fibers that are normally unresponsive to noxious stimuli ('silent' or 'sleeping' nociceptors) can be 'awakened' by inflammatory substances to contribute to pain and hyperalgesia. According to whether or not tissue inflammation is present, nociceptive pain can be subdivided into inflammatory (eg, pain following a superficial burn) or noninflammatory (eg, pain from a pinprick or pinch) pain, respectively. In addition, nociceptive pain can be broadly subdivided according to anatomic location:

- *Somatic* pain, or musculoskeletal pain, arises from tissues such as the skin, mucosa, muscles, joints, bones, and ligaments.
- *Visceral* pain arises from organs such as the bowel, bladder, or ovaries; visceral pain is mediated by specific receptors for stretch, inflammation, or ischemia.

Nociceptive pain is generally responsive to medications such as acetaminophen, nonsteroidal anti-inflammatory drugs (NSAIDs), and opioids.

Note the distinction between 'nociception' and 'pain' or 'nociceptive pain'. Nociception is defined as the stimulation of specialized nerve fibers by noxious stimuli – but it is the somatosensory cortex that consciously perceives the sensations as 'pain'.

Neuropathic pain

In 1994, the International Association for the Study of Pain (IASP) defined neuropathic pain as *"pain caused by a lesion or dysfunction of the nervous system"* [2]. This definition has, however, outgrown its meaning. *"Neuropathic pain"* is in need for an up-to-date re-definition and reclassification, due to our recent scientific and clinical understanding of the mechanisms and manifestations of neuropathic and inflammatory pain disorders.

Neuropathic pain is due to pathologic changes in the neuronal pain pathways. The pain signal is maintained ectopically by a dysfunction in the activity of tissue nociceptors and/or by abnormal pain circuits in the CNS.

According to whether or not inflammation is present and affects the peripheral pain pathways, neuropathic pain can be further subdivided into inflammatory pain (eg, cancer pain, herpes zoster neuritis or shingles, complex regional pain syndrome) or noninflammatory pain (eg, postherpetic neuralgia, trigeminal neuralgia, stump pain).

Of importance are the diagnostic criteria for neuropathic pain. These are:

- a medical history indicating a lesion or disease in the nervous system
- pain distribution corresponding to the innervation territory of a peripheral nerve, nerve root, or CNS structure
- sensory disturbances (evoked or spontaneous) in the pain area

Most neuropathic pain conditions develop after partial injuries to the peripheral nervous system. Recent findings suggest that a number of diffusible factors might be involved in causing a 'neuropathic spin' in some pain states (eg, cancer pain and other pathologic inflammatory pain conditions). For example, as observed in animal models of partial nerve injury, both injured and uninjured primary sensory neurons acquire the ability to express genes *de novo* and, therefore, change their phenotype (*phenotypic shift*). Tissue-related growth factors (eg, nerve growth factor [NGF]), in combination with specific proinflammatory cytokines (eg, tumor necrosis factor [TNF]-α, interleukin [IL]-1β), might not only sensitize tissue nociceptors, but also generate ectopic and spontaneous activity in these small nerve fibers.

One example is the upregulation or induction of catecholamine receptors in undamaged nociceptors; in this condition, nociceptors are activated by norepinephrine, and the resulting neuropathic pain has been called *sympathetically maintained pain*. Reversal of the phenotypic shift is associated with a reduction in neuropathic pain.

There is considerable hope that the identification of the diffusible factors causing altered gene expression in the dorsal root ganglia sensory neurons will direct research to discover more effective treatments. Early and aggressive pain interventions, and the use of specific therapies that disengage gene expression, might be sufficient to uncouple the phenotypic shift and reverse a difficult pain syndrome into an easy-to-treat condition.

Neuropathic pain is typically described as shooting, stabbing, burning, or searing. It is relatively insensitive to NSAIDs, but may be responsive to other classes of drugs, such as antidepressants, anticonvulsants, and opioids.

The processing of pain

The processing of pain information is complex, but it can be broken down into a number of key stages. These are:

- transduction
- transmission to the spinal cord
- spinal cord processing
- ascending pathways to and processing by the brain
- descending pathways

Nociceptors (transduction)

Nociceptors are specialized free nerve endings situated at the distal end of sensory neurons of Aδ fiber and C fiber type. They are stimulated by noxious chemical, mechanical, and thermal stimuli [2,3].

The stimulation of nociceptors, leading to depolarization, is a process in which numerous chemicals participate [4]. For example, the identification of prostaglandins (PGs) has led to an understanding of the action of aspirin and other NSAIDs that inhibit the formation of PGs, namely PGE_2 [5].

Transmission to the spinal cord

Pain impulses are conducted to the dorsal horn of the spinal cord by two types of nociceptor fibers:

- Aδ fibers – these are thinly myelinated fibers, sometimes referred to as 'fast pain fibers' [3].
- C fibers – these are unmyelinated fibers ('slow pain fibers') that have a lower conduction velocity than Aδ fibers.

The activation of Aδ fibers has been associated with the initial sharp, pricking pain ('first pain'), while the activation of C fibers has been associated with the later burning, dull, or aching pain ('second pain') [3,6].

Spinal cord processing

The Aδ and C fibers enter the spinal cord (see **Figure 1**). Here, the Aδ fibers terminate in lamina I, while the C fibers terminate in lamina II (the substantia gelatinosa, a system of densely interconnecting neurons in the dorsal horn) and lamina V.

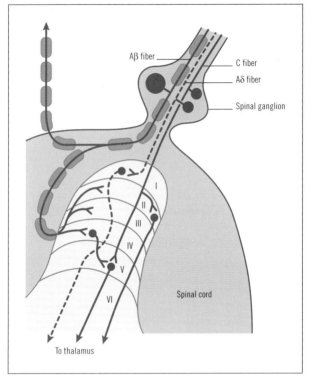

Figure 1. Spinal cord processing.

Reproduced with permission from Springer-Verlag (Mense SS. Functional neuroanatomy for pain stimuli. Reception, transmission, and processing. *Schmerz* 2004;18:225–37).

Ascending pathways to the brain

The nociceptive pathway that transmits pain information to the cerebral cortex is made up of a sequence of three neurons (see **Figure 2**).

- The first-order neuron has its cell body in the dorsal root ganglion, and projects to peripheral tissue and the dorsal horn of the spinal cord.
- The second-order neuron, synapsing with the first-order neuron, crosses over and ascends the contralateral spinal cord. There are several ascending pathways, including

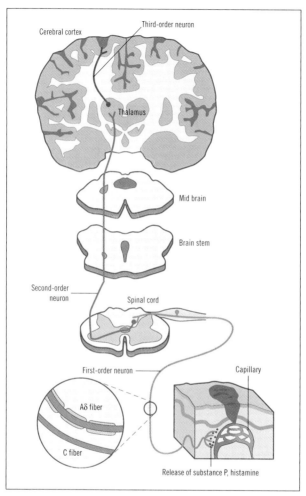

Figure 2. Ascending pathways to the brain. The lateral spinothalamic tract is a major pathway for the transmission of nociceptive stimuli to the brain. The Aδ and C fibers cross and ascend the spinal cord in the anterolateral quadrant. The nociceptive fibers have two regions of the thalamus as their destination: the lateral nucleus and the medial nucleus. Axons that terminate in the thalamus synapse with third-order neurons. These, projecting to topographically organized regions of the somatosensory cortex, enable the pain to be localized.

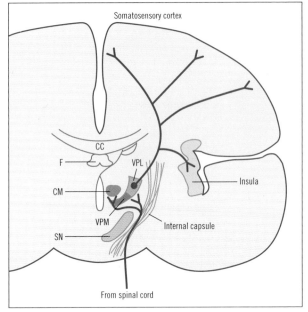

Figure 3. Some central structures involved in pain processing. The figure illustrates thalamic structures likely to receive cardiac pain input from the spinothalamic tract, with projections to the somatosensory cortex. CC: corpus callosum; CM: centromedian and other intralaminar nuclei; F: fornix; SN: substantia nigra; VPL: ventroposterior lateral nucleus; VPM: ventroposterior medial nucleus.

Reproduced with permission from the National Institutes of Health *(Interactive Textbook on Clinical Symptom Research.* Available from: http://symptomresearch.nih.gov/chapter_25/sec11/crfs11pg1.htm).

the spinothalamic tract (a major pain signaling pathway), the spinoreticular tract, and the spinomesencephalic tract, which has a major role in determining the quality and intensity of pain [7]. The second-order neuron is sometimes referred to as the T (transmission) neuron.

- The third-order neuron projects from the thalamus to the basal ganglia, limbic system, and cerebral cortex.

Processing by the brain

Figure 3 and **Table 1** set out the principal brain structures involved in processing pain information.

Brain area	Key roles
Reticular formation	Cluster of neurons in the brain stem
	Rich sensory input
	Role in evaluation of pain stimuli, including affective, motivational, and autonomic aspects
Thalamus	Central importance in pain perception and evaluation
	Fibers project to the sensory cortex and frontal lobes; the latter are important in behavioral or affective components of pain
	The periaqueductal grey area, the medial portion of the thalamus, has a major role in pain transmission and is rich in opioid receptors; it is considered to be one of the main sites of action of endogenous and exogenous opioids
Hypothalamus	Mediates the autonomic and neuroendocrine responses to pain, eg, activation of the sympathetic autonomic system and the hypothalamic–pituitary–adrenal cortex system, leading to 'fight or flight' reactions (sweating, pallor, increased heart rate)
Limbic system	Sometimes referred to as the 'emotional' brain
	The amygdalae and insula region are key components, and are thought to play an important part in affective and emotional responses to pain
Cerebellum	Has a major part in perception of both the emotional and the sensorimotor (eg, pain associated with movement) components of pain
Cerebral cortex	
Anterior cingulate cortex	Appears to play a part in integrating information about pain perception; this might include evaluating danger and planning avoidance
	Opioid receptors are abundant in this area
Somatosensory cortex	Located in the parietal lobes
	Responsible for the conscious perception of pain
	Evaluates the location and quality of pain

Table 1. Central pain processing.

Descending pathways

Fibers from descending pathways originate in the reticular formation, periaqueductal grey matter, and raphe nuclei [8,9]. Important neurotransmitters are endogenous opioids, serotonin, and norepinephrine. The descending system has mainly been associated with the inhibition of pain

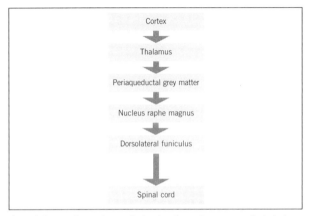

Figure 4. Descending pathways. Antinociceptive pathways are activated when pain signals in the spinothalamic tract reach the brain stem and thalamus. The periaqueductal grey matter and nucleus raphe magnus release endorphins and enkephalins. This leads to the inhibition of nociceptive transmission in the spinal cord.

(see **Figure 4**), but there is now evidence that descending pathways might also have a facilitatory function. It has been suggested that an adverse shift in the balance between inhibition and facilitation contributes significantly to chronic pain conditions [10].

Chronic pain

"The most important clinical development in chronic pain during the last decade has not been new treatments but a thoroughly revised interpretation of the mechanisms that act to maintain pain. Pain is no more seen as a predetermined result of simple activation of certain neural structures. It is now understood to be a dynamic phenomenon due to myriad pathophysiological changes in the peripheral and central nervous system in response to disease, injury, or loss of function" [11].

Peripheral nervous system
Phenotype switch of nociceptors
Ectopic activity in damaged axons
Abnormal firing of dorsal root ganglion cells
Unmasking of silent nociceptors
Collateral sprouting
Invasion of dorsal root ganglia by sympathetic postganglionic fibers
Central nervous system
Central sensitization
Microglial activation
Loss of inhibitory interneuron function
Abnormal central nervous system reorganization

Table 2. Pathophysiological mechanisms of chronic pain [11].

Chronic pain has traditionally been defined as pain that lasts for >3 months without any biological value [12]. Chronic pain is not simply acute pain that persists. Acute pain ordinarily has a useful purpose, such as signaling danger or that something is wrong. By contrast, chronic pain has no such value, but is a disease in its own right, causing widespread suffering, distress, and disability.

Critically, chronic pain is associated with long-term changes at every level in the pain system; these changes may, at least in experimental models, be initiated within a very short time frame, often in a matter of hours. Some of the multiple mechanisms that underlie chronic pain are listed in **Table 2**, and are expanded upon in the next section.

In current pain therapy, the most effective medications still come from the traditional drug groups, some of which have been in use for up to 1,000 years – such as morphine derivatives, NSAIDs, and local anesthetics. Even with recent developments in these and other areas, however, chronic pain remains substantially undertreated.

Development of pain: peripheral nervous system targets

TRPV channels

The transient receptor potential vanilloid (TRPV) 1, 2, and 3 channels are activated by noxious heat, low pH, and capsaicin. Activation of TRPV channels causes nociceptive neurons to 'fire' and leads to the release of neuropeptides, including substance P. On endothelial cells, substance P binds to the neurokinin-1 receptor and promotes the extravasation of plasma into the interstitial tissue. Neuropeptides can activate several other cells, including mast cells; mast cells are known to produce, store, and release NGF (see later) and proinflammatory cytokines.

$\alpha_2\delta$ subunit of neuronal calcium channels

The gabapentinoids, gabapentin and pregabalin, bind with high affinity to the $\alpha_2\delta$ subunit of the voltage-gated calcium channels and produce a decrease in intracellular calcium influx. Gabapentinoids probably produce their analgesic effects by modulating the activity of the $\alpha_2\delta$ subunit [13,14].

Sodium channels

Chronic inflammation results in upregulation of the expression of both tetrodotoxin-resistant (TTX-R) and tetrodotoxin-sensitive (TTX-S) voltage-gated sodium channels. Primary nociceptive sensory neurons express multiple voltage-gated sodium channels.

Observations suggest that the TTX-S (v) 1.7 sodium channel may play a role in pathologic pain. For example, recent studies have shown that a neuropathic pain disorder (familial erythromelalgia) is a channelopathy caused by mutations in the gene encoding the TTX-S (v) 1.7 sodium channel. Familial erythromelalgia is an autosomal dominant disease characterized by severe burning pain in the distal extremities. The pain is typically relieved by cold temperature or ice-pack application to the painful extremities; warm environments and physical exercise aggravate the pain.

TrkA receptors activated by NGF

Mast cells, several immune-inflammatory cells, and endothelial cells synthesize NGF. The NGF receptor, tyrosine kinase A (TrkA) receptor, is expressed by nociceptors. The TrkA–NGF complex is internalized and retrogradely transported to the dorsal root ganglia sensory neuron cell body. Here, it initiates gene transcription that gives rise to the upregulation of multiple receptors and ion channels, and the release of neuropeptides involved in pain transmission. The sensory innervation of cortical and trabecular bone, as well as bone marrow, is extensive, and primarily consists of TrkA-expressing fibers. New evidence indicates that NGF plays an important role in cancer-related bone pain; antibodies directed against NGF are effective in reducing pain in animal models of cancer-induced bone pain [15,16].

Purine receptors

The purine receptors (P2X3, P2X2/3) are activated by ATP, upon which nociceptive sensory nerve fibers are activated and neuropeptides released. P2X3 receptors are localized on peripheral sensory afferents; their activation causes nociception, and contributes to hyperalgesia and mechanical allodynia.

PAR-2 receptors

Proteinase-activated receptor (PAR)-2 is activated by mast cell-derived tryptase and other proteinases. PAR-2 receptors are present in primary sensory neurons and might be involved in mechanisms of hyperalgesia.

Bradykinin receptors

The bradykinin receptors (B1, B2) are activated by bradykinin. Nociceptive sensory neurons express the bradykinin receptors B1 and B2; expression of B1 receptors is induced by tissue injury, and B1 contributes significantly to inflammatory hyperalgesia.

Development of pain: central nervous system targets [17]

Neurokinin-1 and NMDA receptors

During nociceptive activity, incoming small-fiber afferents release neuropeptides (substance P, calcitonin gene-related peptide, cholecystokinin, neurokinin-A) and excitatory amino acids (EAAs) (glutamate, aspartate) within the dorsal horn. Neuropeptides and EAAs can cause transient depolarization of the dorsal horn pain-transmitting neurons (PTNs) by acting on specific receptors. Neurokinin-1 receptors are activated by substance P, while N-methyl-D-aspartate (NMDA) and α-amino-3-hydroxy-5-methyl-4-isoxazole-propionic acid (AMPA), kainate, and the metabotropic receptors are activated by EAAs.

NMDA receptors seem to have a role in pain modulation. These receptors are normally inoperative because of the Mg^{2+}-blocking effect; however, the intense and/or prolonged 'barrage' by substance P and EAAs causes the removal of the Mg^{2+} block from the NMDA receptor. The resulting Ca^{2+} influx causes a series of intracellular changes (including production of nitric oxide) and prolonged sensitization of the PTNs (central sensitization).

Microglia

Increasing evidence suggests that, as a consequence of inflammation of and/or trauma to peripheral nerves, dorsal horn PTN hyperexcitability is dramatically amplified via spinal cord microglia activation. It is still unclear what activates the microglia in the spinal cord; however, neuron-to-glia signals appear to play a role. These include specific substances called *fractalkines* (proteins in the chemokine family), which are expressed on the extracellular surface of the PTNs' sensory afferents. In specific pathologic states or conditions, fractalkines detach from neurons and bind to activate nearby microglia.

Several lines of evidence indicate an emerging role for microglia-derived p38 mitogen-activated protein kinase (MAPK) in the development of pathologic pain. In microglia, p38 MAPK promotes the synthesis and release of proinflammatory cytokines, including TNF-α, IL-1β, and IL-6. Microglia activation also leads to an increase in the production of PGs, nitric oxide, EAAs, ATP, and reactive oxygen species.

References

1.   Pain terms: a list with definitions and notes on usage. Recommended by the IASP Subcommittee on Taxonomy. *Pain* 1979;6:249.

2.   Merskey H, Bogduk N, Editors. *Classification of Chronic Pain. Description of Chronic Pain Syndromes and Definitions of Pain Terms*, 2nd edn. Seattle: IASP Press, 1994.

3.   Barasi S. The physiology of pain. *Surg Nurse* 1991;4:14–20.

4.   McHugh JM, McHugh WB. Pain: neuroanatomy, chemical mediators, and clinical implications. *AACN Clin Issues* 2000;11:168–78.

5.   Woolf CJ, Salter MW. Neuronal plasticity: Increasing the gain in pain. *Science* 2000;288:1765–8.

6.   Johnson BW. Pain mechanisms: anatomy, physiology and neurochemistry. In: Raj PP, Editor. *Practical Management of Pain*, St Louis: Mosby, 2000:117–44.

7.   Heavner JE, Willis WD. Pain pathways: anatomy and physiology. In: Raj PP, Editor. *Practical Management of Pain*, 3rd edn. St Louis: Mosby, 2000:107–16.

8   Westlund KN. Neurophysiology of nociception. In: Pappagallo M, Editor. *The Neurological Basis of Pain*. New York: McGraw-Hill, 2005:3–19.

9.   Wilcox GL, et al. Pharmacology of pain transmission and modulation. In: Pappagallo M, Editor. *The Neurological Basis of Pain*. New York: McGraw-Hill, 2005:31–52.

10. Ren K, Dubner R. Descending modulation in persistent pain: an update. *Pain* 2002;100:1–6.

11. Nurmikko TJ, Nash TP, Wiles JR. Recent advances: control of chronic pain. *BMJ* 1998;317:1438–41.

12. International Association for the Study of Pain, Subcommittee on Taxonomy. Classification of chronic pain. Descriptions of chronic pain syndromes and definitions of pain terms. *Pain Suppl* 1986;3:S1–226.

13. Gee NS, Brown JP, Dissanayake VU, et al. The novel anticonvulsant drug, gabapentin (Neurontin), binds to the alpha2delta subunit of a calcium channel. *J Biol Chem* 1996;271:5768–76.

14. Dooley DJ, Donovan CM, Meder WP, et al. Preferential action of gabapentin and pregabalin at P/Q-type voltage-sensitive calcium channels: inhibition of K$^+$-evoked [3H]-norepinephrine release from rat neocortical slices. *Synapse* 2002;45:171–90.

15. Sevcik MA, Ghilardi JR, Peters CM, et al. Anti-NGF therapy profoundly reduces bone cancer pain and the accompanying increase in markers of peripheral and central sensitization. *Pain* 2005;115:128–41.

16. Halvorson KG, Kubota K, Sevcik MA, et al. A blocking antibody to nerve growth factor attenuates skeletal pain induced by prostate tumor cells growing in bone. *Cancer Res* 2005;65:9426–35.

17. Pappagallo M, Shaiova L, Perlov E, et al. Difficult pain syndromes: bone pain, visceral pain, neuropathic pain. In: Berger AM, Shuster JL, Von Roenn JH, Editors. *Principles and Practice of Palliative Pain and Supportive Oncology*. Philadelphia: Lippincott Williams & Wilkins, 2006.

2 • Epidemiology of chronic pain

Adults

Prevalence and incidence

Chronic pain is a significant national public health problem. It is the most frequent reason for individuals to seek medical care, and accounts for millions of medical visits annually. The American Pain Society's 'Chronic Pain in America' survey has estimated that 9% of the adult population suffers from moderate to severe, noncancer-related pain [1]. Two-thirds of these people say that they have been living with the pain for >5 years. Pain was found to have a significant impact on quality of life and emotional wellbeing, with patients experiencing significant improvements in these factors when their pain was well controlled. In hospitalized patients, pain is associated with an increased recovery time and length of stay, as well as worse treatment outcomes, all of which have healthcare quality and cost implications [2,3].

Chronic pain is highly prevalent in all countries that have been studied, with no striking national differences.

North America
- Overall, approximately 30% of the US population have experienced chronic pain at some point in their lives. Chronic pain is one of the most common causes of

long-term disability, partially or totally disabling some 50 million people [4,5].
- In a US survey among health organization members (n=1,016), 45% reported recurrent or persistent pain. This was severe, with substantial activity limitation, in 8% [6].
- The 2000–2001 Canadian Community Health Survey (n=125,574) found that 18% of women and 14% of men suffered from chronic pain. This was comparable with previous studies in Canada [7].

Europe
- A 2005, large-scale, computer-assisted telephone interview study in 15 European countries and Israel (n=46,394) identified individuals who:
  - had suffered from pain for at least 6 months
  - had experienced pain in the last month
  - had experienced pain at least twice a week
  - rated their pain intensity, when they last experienced pain, as at least 5 on a 10-point numeric rating scale (where 1 = no pain at all and 10 = the worst pain imaginable)

The researchers found that 19% of respondents fulfilled all of the above four criteria; 34% of these had severe pain and 66% had moderate pain [8]. Other European studies have found rates of chronic pain in the region of 15–30% [9,10].

Australia
- In a 1998 study of randomly selected respondents aged ≥18 years (n=2,092), 22.1% reported chronic pain [11].

Other countries
Rates from smaller studies are again broadly comparable with those quoted above, eg:
- 20% prevalence of headache among Indian children and adolescents [12]

- 23% prevalence of low back pain (LBP) among Indian manual workers [13]
- 28% prevalence of LBP among Tunisian schoolchildren [14]

Pain in children and adolescents is discussed further later in this chapter.

Age

Most studies have found that the prevalence of chronic pain increases with age, especially for certain pain syndromes, eg, joint pain, chronic widespread pain, and fibromyalgia [15]. Common age-related pain problems include:

- pain from arthritis
- back pain
- pain following shingles (herpes zoster)
- pain following stroke
- cancer pain
- visceral pain

Health professionals who deal with older people stress, however, that pain is not a 'natural' part of growing old, but is often due to treatable conditions. Even more so than among younger patients, pain among the elderly is substantially underassessed and undertreated. Older patients are also, generally, underrepresented in pain clinic populations [16].

Gender

Review of the literature on sex-prevalence ratios (prevalence in females versus prevalence in males) reveals a higher prevalence for females for the following conditions: headache, migraine, temporomandibular pain, burning mouth pain, neck pain, shoulder pain, back pain, knee pain, abdominal pain, and fibromyalgia [15]. Overall, there is a female predominance for chronic pain (see **Figure 1**). However, this is not large, and it is often less important than factors such as age and economic circumstances [17].

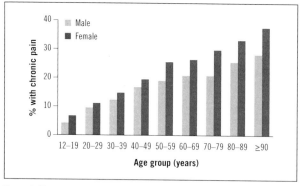

Figure 1. The prevalence of chronic pain by age and gender, Canada.

Reproduced with permission from Statistics Canada (*CCHS, 2000–2001*. Available from: www.biomedcentral.com/1472-6874/4/s1/s17/figure/F3. Accessed August 30, 2007).

Ethnicity

The issue of ethnic disparity regarding health and treatment is complex. People of different ethnic/racial origins have different health patterns. In addition to genetics and clinician bias, cultural differences exist regarding the use of available healthcare. For instance, while older African Americans are more likely than whites to rate their health as poor, they are less likely to use formal health service agencies [18]. Physicians need to be aware of these cultural influences. In the course of developing a pain management plan, physicians should conduct culturally sensitive pain assessments that elicit information regarding the beliefs of the patient and his/her family regarding the pain experience and approaches toward healing practices [19].

Cleeland et al. found that patients treated at centers that predominantly cared for minorities were three times more likely to have inadequate pain management than those treated elsewhere [20]. However, the differences in pain levels cannot be explained entirely by treatment differences. In a 2005 study, African Americans reported greater pain-related interference with daily living, although African Americans and Caucasians did not differ significantly with regard to pain prevalence or severity [21].

History of injury (38% in one study)
Nontraumatic health problems (eg, cardiac disease)
Less formal education
Lower socioeconomic status
Poor housing conditions; living in rented accommodation
Unemployment
Depression (estimates of prevalence range from 31% to 100%, and pain complaints in depressed patients range from 34% to 66%)
Reduced social support; domestic discord
Certain occupations (eg, farmers, blue-collar workers)
Higher body mass index among females
Being retired

Table 1. Factors associated with chronic pain [4,9–11,17].

Other associations

A number of additional factors are associated with an increased risk of chronic pain (see **Table 1**) [4,9–11,17]. The most consistent associations in community studies have been with sustained injury, concomitant health problems, and lower socioeconomic status (see **Figure 2**) [22].

Type/site of pain

The most common disorders that cause chronic pain are diseases of the musculoskeletal and connective tissue systems [9–11].

Functional impairment

Chronic pain has a high impact on the sufferer's day-to-day function, and a range of activities are often severely curtailed. Studies have reported difficulties with daily chores, social life, and work, and a higher rate of unemployment among chronic pain sufferers [11,23–25]. Breivik et al. observed that 19% of patients had lost their job because of chronic pain [8]. Chronic pain sufferers also have low scores for quality of life [10,26].

LBP is one of the most common causes of functional impairment (see **Chapter 4**). The third National Health and Nutrition Examination Survey (NHANES III) estimated during a 12-month

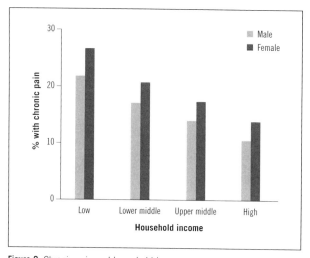

Figure 2. Chronic pain and household income.

period the prevalence of back pain episodes lasting for at least 1 month was 17.8% [27]. Americans spend at least $50 billion each year on LBP – it is the most common cause of job-related disability and second only to the common cold as a cause of work absences in adults aged <45 years [28,29].

> "The 'chronic' in chronic pain encapsulates the sense of defeatism that characterizes the common attitude of many patients and healthcare providers who are dealing with this perplexing and debilitating problem" [17].

Healthcare utilization

Not surprisingly, chronic pain sufferers are heavy users of healthcare services, often presenting with multiple or unexplained symptoms. Many patients also attend alternative practitioners (often without informing their healthcare practitioner) (see **Figure 3**) [30], and a high proportion take prescription or over-the-counter medications. Studies indicate that only 2–5% of chronic pain sufferers have been evaluated or treated by a pain specialist [8,31].

Economic costs

Chronic pain extracts a high cost both from healthcare systems and from society in general. The estimated economic costs for LBP alone have ranged from $20 to $50 billion per year, while the direct medical costs for outpatient visits related to chronic pelvic pain have been estimated at $881.5 million per year [24]. The economic costs for chronic pain in general have been estimated at $86.2 billion per year [32].

A cross-sectional study, based on survey data from 28,902 working adults in the USA, was reported in 2003 [33]. This study found that 13% of the workforce had experienced a loss of productivity during a 2-week period due to a common pain condition (arthritis, back, headache, or other musculoskeletal).

In monetary terms, this loss of productivity was calculated to cost $61.3 billion, with $14.4 billion due to absenteeism and the rest due to the survey participants being at work, but with impaired productivity due to the pain. The authors also commented that this might be an underestimation, as those chronic pain patients who remain employed may adjust both their performance and the perception of their performance over time.

Children and adolescents

Chronic and recurrent pain in children and adolescents has a point prevalence of approximately 15%, with girls reporting more pain than boys, and incidence peaking at an average of 14 years of age [34]. The most common complaint is headache, followed by recurrent abdominal pain and musculoskeletal pain. Studies examining pain in American children are unfortunately lacking; however, chronic pain has been consistently found to be a common problem among children and adolescents in many other countries [34–37]. **Table 2** lists

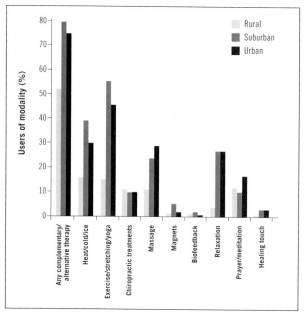

Figure 3. Complementary/alternative modalities used by study participants for the self-treatment of pain: Michigan, June 2000–June 2002 (n=595). In addition, 28% of study participants took herbal products and supplements [30].

the chronic pain symptoms and related disabilities that were found in a 2005 German study among 749 schoolchildren (aged 6–18 years) [38].

As in adults, chronic pain in childhood is frequently associated with medical conditions. **Table 3** shows the results from a study of 207 children (mean age 13.1 years) who were attending a pain referral center [39]. Concomitant medical conditions were present in 51% of the children. In 62 children (30%), however, no organic disorder was found. The most common symptoms in this group were headache, multiple pains, and limb pains. Pain-associated problems and disabilities were common.

	Percentage
Pain present for >6 months:	30.8
Among these:	
Headache	60.5
Abdominal pain	43.3
Limb pain	33.6
Back pain	32.0
Pain caused:	
Sleep problems	60.5
Inability to pursue hobbies	43.3
Eating problems	33.6
School absence	32.0
Inability to meet friends	46.7
Pain perceived as triggered by:	
Weather conditions	33.0
Illness	30.7
Physical exertion	21.9
50.9% had sought professional help and 51.5% were using medications	

Table 2. Chronic pain in schoolchildren (aged 6–18 years) [38].

Condition	Number of children
Cerebral palsy/spasticity	22
Malignant tumors	18
Scoliosis	11
Benign tumors	7
Cystic fibrosis	6
Fibromyalgia	5
Intellectual delay	4
Talipes equinovarus or flat feet	4
Vertebral or spinal cord abnormalities	4
Other	33

Table 3. Concomitant medical conditions in children (mean age 13.1 years) with chronic pain.

Reproduced with permission from Australasian Medical Publishing (Chalkiadis GA. Management of chronic pain in children. *Med J Aust* 2001;175:476–9).

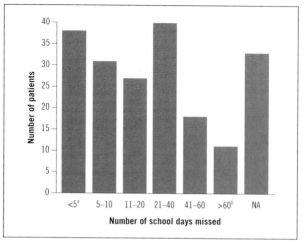

Figure 4. School days missed by children (mean age 13.1 years) due to chronic pain (n=207). ªNine children did not miss any days. ᵇSeven children no longer attended school because of their pain. NA: not applicable (patients were unable to attend school because of a concomitant condition or because they were not of school age).

Reproduced with permission from Australasian Medical Publishing (Chalkiadis GA. Management of chronic pain in children. *Med J Aust* 2001;175:476-9).

These included:

- school absences (95%) (see **Figure 4**)
- inability to participate in sport (71%)
- sleep disruption (71%)

All in all, chronic pain among children is common and is frequently associated with physical illness and substantial disability, as in adults. A particular issue in relation to children, however, is that bullying, sexual or physical abuse, parental disharmony, and difficulties at school may all contribute to abnormal pain behavior. These possibilities need to be investigated in each individual child, and addressed in both management and research [35].

References

1. Roper Starch Worldwide for the American Academy of Pain Medicine, American Pain Society, and Janssen Pharmaceutica. *Chronic Pain in America: Roadblocks to Relief*, 1999.

2. Pavlin DJ, Chen C, Penaloza DA, et al. Pain as a factor complicating recovery and discharge after ambulatory surgery. *Anesth Analg* 2002;95:627–34.

3. Pavlin DJ, Rapp SE, Polissar NL, et al. Factors affecting discharge time in adult outpatients. *Anesth Analg* 1998;87:816–26.

4. Elliott AM, Smith BH, Penny KI, et al. The epidemiology of chronic pain in the community. *Lancet* 1999;354:1248–52.

5. Brookoff D. Chronic pain: 1. A new disease? *Hosp Pract (Minneap)* 2000;35:45–52,59.

6. Von Korff M, Dworkin SF, Le Resche L. Graded chronic pain status: an epidemiologic evaluation. *Pain* 1990;40:279–91.

7. Interior Health. *Preliminary Analysis of the Canadian Community Health Survey*, 2002. Available from: www.interiorhealth.ca. Accessed July 6, 2007.

8. Breivik H, Collett B, Ventafridda V, et al. Survey of chronic pain in Europe: prevalence, impact on daily life, and treatment. *Eur J Pain* 2006;10:287–333.

9. Magni G, Marchetti M, Moreschi C, et al. Chronic musculoskeletal pain and depressive symptoms in the National Health and Nutrition Examination. I. Epidemiologic follow-up study. *Pain* 1993;53:163–8.

10. Andersson HI, Ejlertsson G, Leden I, et al. Chronic pain in a geographically defined general population: studies of differences in age, gender, social class, and pain localization. *Clin J Pain* 1993;9:174–82.

11. Blyth FM, March LM, Cousins MJ. Chronic pain-related disability and use of analgesia and health services in a Sydney community. *Med J Aust* 2003;179:84–7.

12. Chakravarty A. Chronic daily headache in children and adolescents: a clinic based study in India. *Cephalalgia* 2005;25:795–800.

13. Sharma SC, Singh R, Sharma AK, et al. Incidence of low back pain in work-age adults in rural North India. *Indian J Med Sci* 2003;57:145–7.

14. Bejia I, Abid N, Ben Salem K, et al. Low back pain in a cohort of 622 Tunisian schoolchildren and adolescents: an epidemiological study. *Eur Spine J* 2005; 14:331–6.

15. LeResche L. Epidemiologic perspectives on sex differences in pain. In: Fillingim RB, Editor. *Sex, Gender and Pain*. Seattle: IASP Press, 2000:233–49.

16. Canadian Psychological Association. *Chronic Pain Among Seniors*. Available from: www.cpa.ca. Accessed July 17, 2006.

17. Meana M, Cho R, DesMeules M. Chronic pain: the extra burden on Canadian women. *BMC Women's Health* 2004;4(Suppl. 1):S17.

18. Green CR, Baker TA, Smith EM, et al. The effect of race in older adults presenting for chronic pain management: a comparative study of black and white Americans. *J Pain* 2003;4:82–90.

19. Breuer B. Epidemiology of pain. In: Pappagallo M, Editor. *The Neurological Basis of Pain*. New York: McGraw-Hill, 2005:179–94.

20. Cleeland CS, Gonin R, Hatfield AK, et al. Pain and its treatment in outpatients with metastatic cancer. *New Engl J Med* 1994;330:592–6.

21. Ruehlman LS, Karoly P, Newton C. Comparing the experiential and psychosocial dimensions of chronic pain in African Americans and Caucasians: findings from a national community sample. *Pain Med* 2005;6:49–60.

22. Statistics Canada. *CCHS, 2000–2001*. Available from: www.biomedcentral.com. Accessed July 6, 2007.

23. Birse TM, Lander J. Prevalence of chronic pain. *Can J Public Health* 1998;89:129–31.

24. Mathias SD, Kuppermann M, Liberman RF, et al. Chronic pelvic pain: prevalence, health-related quality of life, and economic correlates. *Obstet Gynecol* 1996; 87:321–7.

25. Smith BH, Elliott AM, Chambers WA, et al. The impact of chronic pain in the community. *Fam Pract* 2001;18:292–9.

26. Strine TW, Hootman JM, Chapman DP, et al. Health-related quality of life, health risk behaviors, and disability among adults with pain-related activity difficulty. *Am J Public Health* 2005;95:2042–8.

27. Dillon C, Paulose-Ram R, Hirsch R, et al. Skeletal muscle relaxant use in the United States: data from the Third National Health and Nutrition Examination Survey (NHANES III). *Spine* 2004;29:892–6.

28. National Institute of Neurological Disorders and Stroke. *Low Back Pain Fact Sheet.* Available from: www.ninds.nih.gov. Accessed July 5, 2007.

29. National Institutes of Health. Your aching back: searching for better pain relief. *NIH News in Health*, May 2005. Available from: http://newsinhealth.nih.gov. Accessed July 5, 2007.

30. Vallerand AH, Fouladbakhsh JM, Templin T. The use of complementary/ alternative medicine therapies for the self-treatment of pain among residents of urban, suburban, and rural communities. *Am J Public Health* 2003;93:923–5.

31. Turk DC. When is a person with chronic pain a patient? *American Pain Society Bulletin*, 2005;15. Available from: www.ampainsoc.org. Accessed July 6, 2007.

32. Turk DC. Clinical effectiveness and cost-effectiveness of treatments for patients with chronic pain. *Clin J Pain* 2002;18:355–65.

33. Stewart WF, Ricci JA, Chee E, et al. Lost productive time and cost due to common pain conditions in the US workforce. *JAMA* 2003;290:2443–54.

34. Goodman JE, McGrath PJ. The epidemiology of pain in children and adolescents: a review. *Pain* 1991;46:247–64.

35. Perquin CW, Hazebroek-Kampschreur AA, Hunfeld JA, et al. Pain in children and adolescents: a common experience. *Pain* 2000;87:51–8.

36. Perquin CW, Hazebroek-Kampschreur AA, Hunfeld JA, et al. Chronic pain among children and adolescents: physician consultation and medication use. *Clin J Pain* 2000;16:229–35.

37. van Dijk A, McGrath PA, Pickett W, et al. Pain prevalence in nine- to 13-year-old schoolchildren. *Pain Res Manag* 2006;11:234–40.

38. Roth-Isigkeit A, Thyen U, Stoven H, et al. Pain among children and adolescents: restrictions in daily living and triggering factors. *Pediatrics* 2005;115:e152–62.

39. Chalkiadis GA. Management of chronic pain in children. *Med J Aust* 2001;175:476–9.

3 • Pain assessment

The accurate assessment of pain is a prime requirement for effective pain control. Diagnosis of the type of pain, its severity, and its effect on the patient is necessary in order to plan appropriate treatments, and is an integral part of the overall clinical assessment.

Pain management standards published by the Joint Commission for the Accreditation of Healthcare Organizations (JCAHO) require that all healthcare organizations that are accredited by JCAHO implement policies and procedures that make pain assessment and effective management strategies a routine part of every patient's care [1].

Why assess?

The main purpose of the assessment (and reassessment) of the patient with pain is to evaluate the effectiveness of the pain management plan. At baseline, clinicians should perform a comprehensive pain assessment in order to diagnose the cause of the pain, and evaluate the multiple dimensions of the pain experience (see **Table 1**). Subsequent evaluations of the effectiveness of the pain management plan often focus on determining whether the intensity of the pain has decreased as a result of pharmacologic and nonpharmacologic interventions [2].

Obtain and review past medical records and diagnostic studies
Obtain a detailed history, including an assessment of the pain characteristics and intensity
Conduct a physical examination, emphasizing the neurologic and musculoskeletal examination
Obtain a psychosocial assessment
Provide an appropriate diagnostic work-up to determine the cause of pain

Table 1. Initial pain assessment.

Reproduced with permission from the American Medical Association (Evans MR. *Pain Management: The Online Series*. AMA, 2005. Available from: www.ama-cmeonline.com).

It has been shown that healthcare professionals tend to underrate the level of pain that a patient is experiencing, and this discrepancy tends to widen as the severity of pain increases [3,4]. Conversely, family members tend to overestimate pain in their relatives [5]. The patient, if cognitively competent and able to communicate, remains the prime and only evaluator of his/her own pain.

When asked about barriers to good pain management in their own practice setting, 76% of physicians cited poor assessment of pain as a problem [6].

What to assess?

Pain is a complex experience. Its assessment should be multidimensional, and should include: medical history; physical examination; assessment of psychosocial, family, and cultural aspects; a record of pain history; and the effect of previous treatments on the patient's pain.

Patient history

The patient's medical history should characterize the pain in detail (location, temporal pattern, quality, intensity, and exacerbating/alleviating factors) [7], and include any medically relevant problems relating to the pain (eg, history of diabetes, infections, gastrointestinal disease, cardiovascular disease, neurologic disorder, medication, alcohol intake). An additional vital descriptive element is the effect that the pain has on the patient's daily working and social activities.

Pain characteristics and intensity

The patient's subjective description of the pain, its quality, and the factors that exacerbate or relieve it are potentially valuable pointers to the source of the pain [7]. Ideally, they will also indicate the optimal etiologic and symptomatic management.

- About two-thirds of cancer patients report episodes of 'breakthrough pain' [8]. This phrase refers to a transitory flare of pain that occurs on a background of persistent pain that is relatively well-controlled with opioids [9]. These flares can be unpredictable or idiopathic. Breakthrough pain is discussed in detail in **Chapter 12**.
- Recurrent pain is often reported by patients with headaches, dysmenorrhea, sickle cell disease, or musculoskeletal disorders.
- Persistent pain syndromes are commonly associated with cancer, nonmalignant progressive diseases (eg, acquired immune deficiency syndrome, connective tissue diseases), and nonprogressive or slowly progressive diseases (eg, severe osteoporosis, painful neuropathy).

> The characteristics of the pain can be valuable pointers towards a diagnosis and optimal management.

Type of pain

Identification of the type of pain is an essential step in making a diagnosis, and a key element in guiding treatment. **Table 2** summarizes the main types of pain and their characteristics.

Assessing pain intensity

The intensity of pain needs to be quantified both as part of the initial pain assessment and on an ongoing basis in order to assess response to treatment. A variety of well-validated pain scales are available. The physician should choose the one

Type of pain	Origin	Characteristics	Pharmacologic treatment
Somatic	Tissues such as skin, joint, muscle, bone, ligament	Typically aching, sharp, or throbbing Often worsened by movement, breathing, and laughing May be constant or intermittent	If somatic pain has an inflammatory mechanism, it should respond to NSAIDs; otherwise use a combination of nonopioid and opioid analgesics
Visceral	Organs such as bowel, bladder, heart, pancreas, uterus	Diffuse, poorly localized, and often intermittent or crampy Often associated with changes in functions such as urination and defecation	Nonopioid and opioid analgesics
Neuropathic	Nerve tissue (eg, from damage, pressure, inflammation)	Typically shooting, stabbing, searing, burning Follows nerve or dermatomal distribution	Responds poorly to NSAIDs Treatment may include a combination of nonopioid and opioid analgesics

Table 2. Types of pain. NSAID: nonsteroidal anti-inflammatory drug.

that is most appropriate to the patient (eg, based on age, comprehension) and apply the method systematically, using it in the same way on each occasion.

Pain assessment tools are either unidimensional or multi-dimensional (taking in composite aspects such as mood, sleep, and the effect of pain on general activity).

Unidimensional pain scales

Common unidimensional pain scales include the numeric rating scale (NRS), the visual analog scale (VAS) (see **Figure 1**), verbal rating scales (VRS), and picture scales. These are all reliable and valid. However, patients tend to prefer NRS and VRS measures over VAS measures [10].

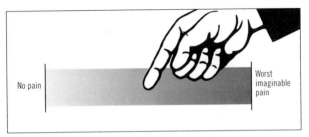

Figure 1. The visual analog scale for pain assessment.

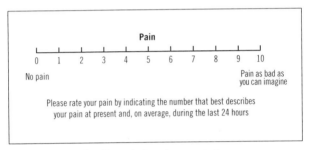

Figure 2. The numeric rating scale for pain assessment.

The NRS is simple to use both at the bedside and in the community. The patient marks the number on a 0–10 line that best describes the intensity of his/her pain. The line should have numbers from 0 to 10, where 0 = 'No pain' and 10 = 'Pain as bad as you can imagine,' accompanied by the instruction: "Please rate your pain by indicating the number that best describes your pain at present and, on average, during the last 24 hours" (see **Figure 2**). Of note, a consensus from a group of experts (the IMMPACT [Initiative on Methods, Measurement, and Pain Assessment in Clinical Trials] consensus) recommends the 11-point (ie, 0–10) NRS measure of pain intensity as a core outcome tool in clinical trials of chronic pain treatments [10].

The faces pain rating scale is widely used in pediatric practice; the example shown in **Figure 3** is one of several versions. It is recommended for children aged ≥3 years, and also in patients

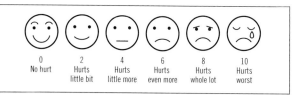

Figure 3. The Wong–Baker Faces Pain Rating Scale.

Reproduced with permission from Elsevier (Wong DL, Hockenberry-Eaton M, Wilson D, et al. *Wong's Essentials of Pediatric Nursing.* Mosby, 2001:1301).

Dimension	Aspects
Biological	Etiology Duration Location Intensity Quality
Affective/psychiatric	Emotional (depression, anxiety) Suffering Psychiatric comorbidities
Cognitive	Meaning of pain Coping strategies Attitudes, beliefs, and knowledge Level of cognition
Behavioral	Pain behaviors Communication of pain
Nonpainful symptoms	Fatigue Sleep Weight changes
Sociocultural	Demographic variables Cultural background Personal, family, and work conditions Caregiver perspective

Table 3. Dimensions of the pain experience.

with cognitive impairment or language barriers [11,12]. This scale is a composite assessment of pain and mood.

Multidimensional pain scales

Multidimensional pain scales have been developed to assess other characteristics of pain more completely, such as the effect

Box 1. Barriers to pain assessment [14,15].

Health professionals who are assessing pain should be vigilant for a number of common difficulties in pain assessment. These include:

- The multidimensional and subjective nature of pain, and the lack of a clearly defined language. The patient may emphasize sensory aspects ("It hurts here"), emotional aspects ("I am so depressed because of the pain"), or functional impairment ("I can hardly get out of bed in the morning"). Further specific questioning may be required to gain a complete picture of how the patient's pain affects his/her life.

- Anxiety or depression.

- Poor communication between patient and health professional:
  - underreporting by the patient
  - underassessment by health professionals or carers
  - language/ethnicity differences
  - reduced cognitive ability
  - reduced level of consciousness
  - knowledge deficit in health professionals regarding pain control

However, assessments in primary care have shown that most physicians and community nurses are keen to enhance their knowledge, skills, and attitudes with regard to pain and symptom control.

of pain on the patient's mood and everyday function. Multiple dimensions of the pain experience are shown in **Table 3**.

The Brief Pain Inventory (BPI) is a multidimensional instrument that was constructed to measure pain caused by cancer and other diseases (eg, rheumatoid arthritis, chronic orthopedic problems). The BPI assesses and quantifies subjective pain intensity (pain worst, pain least, pain average, and pain right now) and the effect of pain on patient function (general activity, mood, ability to walk, normal work, socializing with others, enjoyment of life, and sleep). It is short and can be used for follow-up assessments [13]. The BPI interference scale provides a reliable and valid measure of the interference of pain with physical functioning. It has been translated and used in multiple countries for the assessment of a variety of chronic pain syndromes [10].

Barriers to the accurate assessment of pain are shown in **Box 1**.

Continuing assessment

An initial full assessment should be followed by a further brief assessment following initiation of treatment and at each contact. It is often helpful for the patient to regularly assess his/her own pain at home, using a simple method such as a pain diary.

The frequency of appointments will depend on the patient's response to treatment and the management plan agreed between the patient and his/her carers and health professionals.

References

1. Berry PH, Dahl JL. The new JCAHO pain standards: implications for pain management nurses. *Pain Manag Nurs* 2000;1:3–12.
2. Miaskowski C. Principles of pain assessment. In Pappagallo M, Editor. *The Neurological Basis of Pain.* New York: McGraw-Hill, 2005.
3. Grossman SA, Sheidler VR, Sweeden K, et al. Correlation of patient and caregiver ratings of cancer pain. *J Pain Symptom Manage* 1991;6:53–7.
4. Field L. Are nurses still underestimating patients' pain postoperatively? *Br J Nurs* 1996;5:778–84.
5. Elliott BA, Elliott TE, Murray DM, et al. Patients and family members: the role of knowledge and attitudes in cancer pain. *J Pain Symptom Manage* 1996;12:209–20.
6. Cleeland CS, Gonin R, Hatfield AK, et al. Pain and its treatment in outpatients with metastatic cancer. *N Engl J Med* 1994;330:592–6.
7. Glajchen M. *Pain Assessment. Topics in Pain Management: A Slide Compendium.* Available from: www.stoppain.org. Accessed July 6, 2007.
8. Caraceni A, Martini C, Zecca E, et al. for the Working Group of an IASP Task Force on Cancer Pain. Breakthrough pain characteristics and syndromes in patients with cancer pain. An international survey. *Palliat Med* 2004;18:177–83.
9. Portenoy RK, Hagen NA. Breakthrough pain: definition, prevalence and characteristics. *Pain* 1990;41:273–81.
10. Dworkin RH, Turk DC, Farrar JT, et al. Core outcome measures for chronic pain clinical trials: IMMPACT recommendations. *Pain* 2005;113:9–19.
11. Bieri D, Reeve RA, Champion GD, et al. The Faces Pain Scale for the self-assessment of the severity of pain experienced by children: development, initial validation, and preliminary investigation for ratio scale properties. *Pain* 1990;41:139–50.
12. Taylor LJ, Herr K. Pain intensity assessment: a comparison of selected pain intensity scales for use in cognitively intact and cognitively impaired African American older adults. *Pain Manag Nurs* 2003;4:87–95.
13. Cleeland CS, Ryan KM. Pain assessment: global use of the Brief Pain Inventory. *Ann Acad Med Singapore* 1994;23:129–38.
14. Foley KM. Pain assessment and cancer pain syndromes. In: Doyle D, Hanks GW, MacDonald N, Editors. *Oxford Textbook of Palliative Medicine*, 2nd edn. Oxford: Oxford University Press, 1998:310–31.
15. Von Roenn JH, Cleeland CS, Gonin R, et al. Physician attitudes and practice in cancer pain management. A survey from the Eastern Cooperative Oncology Group. *Ann Intern Med* 1993;119:121–6.

4 • Low back pain syndrome

Low back pain (LBP) (for definition, see **Box 1**) is a large cause of functional impairment [1]. It is the most common cause of job-related disability, and second only to the common cold as a cause of work absences in adults aged <45 years [2,3]. It therefore imposes a huge socioeconomic burden in the USA, with estimated costs ranging from $50 billion to >$100 billion/year [3–5].

Epidemiology

Incidence and prevalence
- Although estimates vary, episodes of LBP that are frequent or persistent have been reported in 15% of the population, with a lifetime prevalence of 65–80% [6].
- The 1-year prevalence of back pain has been reported to be 10–56% [6].
- In North Carolina, chronic LBP has been reported to affect 3.9% of the population, with 34% of these considering themselves permanently disabled and 52% assessing their overall health as only fair to poor [7].

Cost and implications
- Many people who have back pain report that it interferes with their daily activities (eg, work, school, leisure pursuits).

Box 1. What is low back pain?

"Low back pain is usually defined as pain, muscle tension, or stiffness localized below the costal margin and above the inferior gluteal folds, with or without leg pain (sciatica). Low back pain is typically classified as being 'specific' or 'nonspecific'. Specific low back pain refers to symptoms caused by a specific pathophysiologic mechanism, such as hernia nucleus pulposus, infection, inflammation, osteoporosis, rheumatoid arthritis, fracture, or tumor. In only about 10% of patients can specific underlying disease be identified. The vast majority of patients (up to 90%) are labeled as having nonspecific low back pain, which is defined as symptoms without clear specific cause, ie, low back pain of unknown origin. Of note, a variety of abnormalities (degenerative disc and vertebral changes) observed on X-ray, computed tomography (CT), and magnetic resonance imaging (MRI) scans are also called nonspecific, because many people without any symptoms also show these abnormalities" [8].

In chronic low back pain (defined as persisting for ≥3 months) there are usually changes due to a range of disease processes. For a full discussion, see www.emedicine.com/neuro/topic516.htm.

- In 2005–2006, the combined annual direct and indirect cost of LBP were estimated at between $50 billion and over $100 billion [3–5].
- LBP is the most common cause of job-related disability and the second most common neurologic ailment in the USA [3–5].
- Every year, approximately 2% of the work force is compensated for back pain secondary to work-related back injuries [9].

Research by Katz has revealed the following figures [4]:

- A total of 5% of Americans miss at least 1 day of work annually due to LBP.
- More than 80% of workers who report an episode of LBP return to work within 1 month, and >90% return within 3 months. However, 5% never return.
- By the time a worker has been out work for 6 months, the likelihood of returning to work is just 50%; by the time a worker has been out of work for 1 year, the likelihood of ever returning to work drops to 25%.

Referred pain
From abdomen (eg, aortic aneurysm), kidney (eg, pyelonephritis, hydronephrosis), ovary (eg, cysts, cancer), pelvis (eg, endometriosis, pelvic inflammatory disease), or bladder (eg, infection)
Degenerative and structural changes
Spondylolisthesis, gross scoliosis/kyphosis
Spinal stenosis and/or radiculopathy
Inflammatory conditions
Ankylosing spondylitis
Polymyalgia rheumatica
Rheumatoid arthritis (rarely a cause of back pain)
Infections
Discitis
Osteomyelitis (bacterial or tuberculous)
Neoplasms
Metastatic disease
Myeloma or other (more rare) primary cancer
Metabolic bone disease
Osteoporosis with compression fractures
Osteomalacia/vitamin D deficiency
Paget's disease

Table 1. Some causes of low back pain.

Abridged with permission from the UK Department of Health (PRODIGY Guidance. *Back Pain – Lower*, 2005. Available from www.prodigy.nhs.uk).

Risk factors

The main risk factors for the onset of nonspecific LBP most often relate to physical aspects of work. They include [6]:

- heavy physical work that involves the lifting and handling of loads
- awkward postures and movements (eg, bending, twisting, static postures)
- whole body vibration

Children and adolescents

Reviews have reported a prevalence for LBP in children and adolescents that approaches that reported for adults, with an annual incidence of about 15%, and with 50% reporting recurrence [6,10]. Few clear risk factors have been identified in children, but children with LBP are more likely to have emotional and conduct problems, and to have other somatic pains [11].

Causes

Table 1 lists some of the causes of LBP. Often, however, no specific underlying cause can be identified, and a serious cause is relatively rare. Some 1% of people presenting with LBP in primary care have a neoplasm, 4% have compression fractures, and 1–3% have a prolapsed disk [12].

Assessment

Many options are available for evaluation and management of LBP (see **Table 2**). However, there has been a poor consensus on its appropriate work-up and management. In the evaluation of patients with chronic LBP, the main objectives are to [12]:

- identify the source of the pain, ie, to identify the few patients who have a serious underlying disorder (see **Table 1**)
- assess the degree of pain and functional limitation
- define the contributing factors where possible
- develop a management strategy
- conduct a focused history and physical examination to help place patients into one of the three following categories:
    - nonspecific or cryptogenic LBP
    - back pain potentially associated with radiculopathy or spinal stenosis
    - back pain potentially associated with another specific spinal or extraspinal cause

The history should include assessment of psychosocial factors.

Patient history

Cancer risk factors (eg, age ≥50 years, history of cancer, unexplained weight loss)

Risk factors for possible spinal infection (eg, IV drug use, immunosuppression, urinary infection)

Signs or symptoms of cauda equina syndrome (eg, urinary retention, saddle anesthesia, unilateral or bilateral sciatica, sensory and motor deficits)

Signs or symptoms of neurologic involvement (eg, numbness or weakness in the legs, sciatica with radiation past the knee)

Psychosocial indications (eg, belief that pain and activity are harmful, depressed mood, problems with claim and compensation, overprotective family or lack of support). Psychosocial indications can be barriers to recovery

Physical examination

Palpation for spinal tenderness

Neuromuscular testing (including ankle dorsiflexion strength, great toe dorsiflexion strength, ankle and knee reflexes, sensory exam with pinprick sensation in the medial, dorsal, and lateral aspects of the foot)

Straight leg raise

Imaging

Lumbar spine X-rays (AP and lateral views) should be considered when the following red flag indicators exist:

- unrelenting night pain or pain at rest (increased incidence of clinically significant pathology)
- history of or suspicion of cancer (rule out metastatic disease)
- fever >38°C (100.4°F) for >48 hours
- osteoporosis
- other systemic diseases
- neuromotor or sensory deficit
- chronic oral steroids
- immunosuppression
- serious accident or injury
- clinical suspicion of ankylosing spondylitis

MRI/CT is indicated in chronic sciatica/radiculopathy if surgery, cancer, or infection are considerations (red flag indications)

Consider blood testing (including CBC and ESR) if there is suspicion of cancer or infection

Pain assessment

Subjective pain rating

Functional assessment

Clinician's objective assessment

Table 2. Recommendations for the evaluation of the patient with chronic back pain [13]. AP: anteroposterior; CBC: complete blood count; CT: computed tomography; ESR: erythrocyte sedimentation rate; IV: intravenous; MRI: magnetic resonance imaging.

Nonspecific low back pain

Approximately ≥90% of patients who present to primary care have nonspecific LBP [14]. 'Nonspecific' or 'cryptogenic' LBP is pain that occurs in the back (axial pain) with no signs of a serious underlying condition (eg, cancer, infection, cauda equina syndrome), spinal stenosis or radiculopathy, or another specific spinal cause (eg, vertebral compression fracture, ankylosing spondylitis). Degenerative changes (disc degeneration, spondylotic changes) seen in imaging studies are usually considered nonspecific as they correlate poorly with symptoms.

Red flags and prognostic factors

The Agency for Healthcare Research and Quality has defined a set of 'red flags' that relate to patients with LBP [15]. Red flags (see **Table 3**) suggest that there might be serious pathology and that further investigation may be warranted. Other indicators (see **Table 4**) relate to prognosis; they are factors that increase the risk of developing or perpetuating chronic pain (ie, chronification) or long-term disability, including work loss – ie, they signal barriers to recovery [16]. The identification of these prognostic factors should lead to appropriate cognitive and behavioral measures.

Management

Recommendations for the management of back pain are set out in **Table 5**. As indicated by the Katz figures [4], there is a compelling rationale for the aggressive treatment of LBP within the subacute period – between 2–4 weeks and 6 months. Those who remain out of work for an increasing length of time have a diminishing probability of ever returning to work and normal health.

Red flags for spine fracture

Major trauma (eg, vehicle accident or fall from a height)

Minor trauma, or even just strenuous lifting, in older or potentially osteoporotic patients

Red flags for cancer or infection

Age >50 years and new back pain, or age <20 years

History of malignancy

Constitutional symptoms (eg, fever, chills, unexplained weight loss)

Recent bacterial infection (eg, urinary tract infection)

IV drug abuse

Immune suppression (eg, from steroids, transplantation, or HIV)

Pain that worsens when supine; severe nighttime pain; thoracic pain

Structural deformity

Red flags for cauda equina syndrome or rapidly progressing neurologic deficit

Saddle anesthesia (loss of sensation in areas that would sit on a saddle)

Recent onset of bladder dysfunction (eg, urine retention, increased urge frequency, overflow incontinence)

Unexpected laxity of the anal sphincter; recent onset of fecal incontinence; perianal/perineal sensory loss

Severe or progressive neurologic deficit in the lower extremities

Major motor weakness: knee extension, ankle plantar eversion, foot dorsiflexion

Table 3. Red flags for patients with low back pain [15].
HIV: human immunodeficiency virus syndrome; IV: intravenous.

Clinical factors

Previous episodes of back pain

Multiple previous musculoskeletal complaints

Psychiatric history

Alcohol, drugs, cigarettes

Pain experience

Rate pain as severe

Maladaptive pain beliefs

Legal issues or compensation

Premorbid factors

Rate job as physically demanding

Believe they will not be working in 6 months

Do not get along with supervisors or coworkers

Near to retirement

Family history of depression

Enabling spouse

Are unmarried or have been married multiple times

Low socioeconomic status

Troubled childhood (abuse, parental death, alcohol use, difficult divorce)

Table 4. Risk factors for chronic disability.

Reproduced with permission from Regents of the University of Michigan (Chiodo A, Alvarez D, Graziano G, et al. *Guidelines for Clinical Care: Acute Low Back Pain*. University of Michigan Health System, 2005).

Medication
Most patients will have tried over-the-counter back pain remedies before seeking physician consultation
Pharmacologic options include acetaminophen, NSAIDs, muscle relaxants, tramadol, antidepressants, anticonvulsants, and opioids
Physical modalities
Beyond the acute phase, the choice of physical modalities is usually patient-specific, given the dearth of high-quality evidence supporting most interventions
Potential therapies include stretching, ice and heat, massage, manipulation, exercise rehabilitation programs, electrical muscle stimulation, work-hardening programs, and acupuncture
After 6 weeks, all approaches seem to have about the same rates of success
Bed rest should be avoided, and patients should be encouraged to return to work and their usual activities as soon as possible
Patients should be educated in proper posture, sitting position, and lifting techniques
Other therapies
Support groups, counseling, addiction therapy, or relaxation therapy can all improve outcomes
Treatment of coincident depression and anxiety can improve pain control
Alternative therapies are potentially of benefit (see **Chapter 17**)
Interventional pain management (see Chapter 17)
Diagnostic facet and nerve blocks
Therapeutic rhizotomies and nerve ablations
Selective joint injections
Epidural injections
Intradiscal distraction therapy
Spinal endoscopy

Table 5. Recommendations for the management of low back pain [17]. NSAID: nonsteroidal anti-inflammatory drug.

References

1. Dillon C, Paulose-Ram R, Hirsch R, et al. Skeletal muscle relaxant use in the United States: data from the Third National Health and Nutrition Examination Survey (NHANES III). *Spine* 2004; 29:892–6.
2. National Institutes of Health. Your aching back: searching for better pain relief. *NIH News in Health*, May 2005. Available from: http://newsinhealth.nih.gov. Accessed July 30, 2007.
3. National Institute of Neurological Disorders and Stroke. *Low Back Pain Fact Sheet.* Available from: www.ninds.nih.gov. Accessed July 30, 2007.
4. Katz JN. Lumbar disc disorders and low-back pain: socioeconomic factors and consequences. *J Bone Joint Surg Am* 2006;88(Suppl. 2):21–4.

5.   Leigh JP, Markowitz SB, Fahs M, et al. Occupational injury and illness in the United States. Estimates of costs, morbidity, and mortality. *Arch Inter Med* 1997;157:1557–68.

6.   Manchikanti L. Epidemiology of low back pain. *Pain Physician* 2000;3:167–92.

7.   Carey TS, Evans A, Hadler N, et al. Care-seeking among individuals with chronic low back pain. *Spine* 1995;20:312–17.

8.   van Tulder, Koes B. Low back pain. In: McMahon SB, Koltzenburg M, Editors. *Wall and Melzack's Textbook of Pain*. London: Churchill Livingstone, 2006:699–708.

9.   Andersson GB. Epidemiological features of chronic low-back pain. *Lancet* 1999;354:581–5.

10. Balague F, Troussier B, Salminen JJ. Non-specific low back pain in children and adolescents: risk factors. *Eur Spine J* 1999;8:429–38.

11. Jones GT, MacFarlane GJ. Epidemiology of low back pain in children and adolescents. *Arch Dis Child* 2005;90:312–16.

12. Speed C. Low back pain. *BMJ* 2004;328:1119–21.

13. Institute for Clinical Systems Improvement (ICSI). *Acute Low Back Pain*. Bloomington: ICSI, 2006. Available from: www.icsi.org. Accessed July 30, 2007.

14. van Tulder MW, Assendelft WJ, Koes BW, et al. Spinal radiographic findings and nonspecific low back pain. A systematic review of observational studies. *Spine* 1997;22:427–34.

15. US Agency for Health Care Policy and Research. *Acute Low Back Pain Problems in Adults: Assessment and Treatment. Quick Reference Guide for Clinicians*. Agency for Health Care Policy and Research, 1994.

16. Chiodo A, Alvarez D, Graziano G, et al. *Guidelines for Clinical Care: Acute Low Back Pain*. University of Michigan Health System, 2005.

17. Rives PA, Douglass AB. Evaluation and treatment of low back pain in family practice. *J Am Board Fam Pract* 2004;17:S23–31.

5 • Osteoarthritis

Osteoarthritis is the most common form of joint disease in the world, and the single most important cause of locomotor disability [1].

- In the Western world, osteoarthritis ranks fourth in health impact among Western women and eighth among men [2].
- Osteoarthritis is second only to ischemic heart disease as a cause of work-related disability in men aged >50 years, and it is the most common arthritic disease resulting in loss of time from work for both men and women [3].

Prevalence rises steeply with age (see **Figure 1**). By the age of 65 years, the majority of people have objective changes in at least one joint, although not everyone is symptomatic; by the age of 75 years, this is true of 80% of people [4]. The disease usually targets the extremities of long bones; although any synovial joint can be affected, the most frequently involved joints are the hand, knee, hip, and spinal facet joints [5,6].

"There is no generally accepted definition of osteo-arthritis, but most would agree that pathologically it is a condition of synovial joints characterized by focal cartilage loss and an accompanying reparative [inflammatory] bone response" [1].

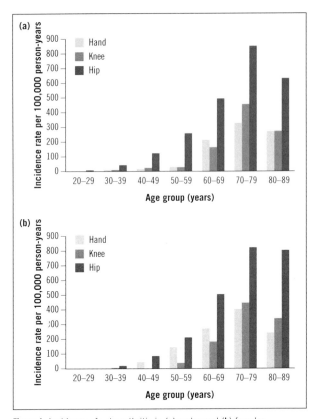

Figure 1. Incidence of osteoarthritis in (**a**) males and (**b**) females.

Reprinted with the permission of Wiley-Liss, Inc., a subsidiary of John Wiley & Sons, Inc. (Oliveria SA, Felson DT, Reed JL, et al. Incidence of symptomatic hand, hip, and knee osteoarthritis among patients in a health maintenance organization. *Arthritis Rheum* 1995;38:1134–41). ©1995 John Wiley & Sons, Inc.

Epidemiology

The etiology of osteoarthritis is multifactorial. **Table 1** sets out the principal risk factors.

A complex disease process

The pathogenesis of osteoarthritis is considered to take place in the following stages [7]:

Risk factor	Comment
Age	The factor most strongly and consistently associated with osteoarthritis; greatest increase is at ages 40–50 years. But the disorder is more complex than a simple age-related degenerative process (see below)
Gender	Women tend to have more multiple joint involvement than men, and a greater prevalence and severity of osteoarthritis of the hands, knees, ankles, and feet
	Men have greater prevalence and severity of osteoarthritis of the hips, wrists, and spine
	Overall, there is a pronounced female preponderance of radiographic evidence for severe osteoarthritic changes, and of symptoms
Ethnicity	Osteoarthritis of the hip is uncommon in black and Indian/Pakistani populations compared with Caucasians, and polyarthritis of the hand is rare in black Africans and Malaysians
	Several other racial differences have also been noted; these are considered to reflect genetic rather than cultural factors
Genetics	A genetic predisposition has often been noted
	Some types appear to be inherited in a Mendelian autosomal pattern
Obesity	The association is inconsistent
	Knee osteoarthritis has been more strongly associated with obesity than hip and ankle arthritis
	Longitudinal studies suggest that obesity in childhood and adolescence is more strongly associated with osteoarthritis than obesity in middle and older age; therefore, obesity may have a long-term effect
Sporting activity	A clear association has not been established; osteoarthritis is, however, more likely to be associated with or to occur following a sporting injury
	High-performance athletes have an increased risk of developing osteoarthrosis
Previous trauma	Patients often give a history of joint injury
Occupation	Results are again inconsistent. Associations have often not been found where they may have been expected, eg, among shipyard workers and pneumatic drill operators. The most consistent risk has been found among agricultural workers, possibly due to heavy lifting and walking over rough ground. An association has also been found with posture (eg, frequent squatting)

Table 1. Risk factors for osteoarthritis [1,5–8].

1. Proteolytic breakdown of the cartilage matrix, with increased production of enzymes that destroy the cartilage matrix. Chondrocytes produce protease inhibitors, but in amounts insufficient to reduce the proteolytic effects.
2. Erosion of the cartilage surface, with release of proteoglycan and collagen fragments into the synovial fluid.
3. Breakdown products of cartilage induce a chronic inflammatory response in the synovium with the release of cytokines and other proinflammatory products. The joint architecture is thereby altered, and compensatory bone overgrowth occurs in an attempt to stabilize the joint. As further mechanical and inflammatory stress occurs on the articular surfaces, the disease continues to progress.

> "Previously considered as a degenerative disease that was an inevitable consequence of aging, osteoarthritis is now viewed as a metabolically dynamic and essentially reparative process that is increasingly amenable to treatment" [1].

Clinical presentation

Pain is the main reason why people with osteoarthritis seek help [2]. Pain can arise from several sites around an osteoarthritic joint, and may be related to increased capsular and interosseous pressure, subchondral microfractures, and bursitis/tendinitis/tenosynovitis secondary to muscle weakness or structural alteration (enthesopathy).

Points to note about the pain are [7]:

- Initially, symptomatic patients experience pain during activity; this can be relieved by rest and may respond to simple analgesics.
- Morning stiffness is common, usually lasting <1 hour.
- Stiffness at rest may develop.
- Pain often increases during the day due to activity.

- Joints may become unstable with disease progression, so that the pain can become more prominent, even at rest, and may fail to respond to medications.

Other common clinical features include [1,7]:

- crepitus
- bony enlargement or deformity
- warmth
- effusion
- muscle weakness or wasting

Assessment

The assessment of arthritis patients should include a complete history and physical examination. In addition, an initial comprehensive assessment of pain should be performed. This should be repeated at regular intervals in order to evaluate the effectiveness of any interventions. Pain assessment should focus on the type and quality of pain, source, intensity, location, duration/time course, pain effect, and effects on personal lifestyle [9].

When possible, self-reporting should be the primary source of pain assessment [9]. Behavioral observations and physiologic measurements may provide additional information, but should not be used as the primary source of pain assessment, except in preverbal children and the cognitively impaired.

Pain is a major cause of disability in people with arthritis. Therefore, the assessment of functional status should be included in the pain assessment. When arthritis pain is persistent or severe, the assessment should include an evaluation of biological, psychological, or social factors that may be contributing to pain, in addition to an assessment of the overall impact of pain on function [9].

Diagnosis is usually supported by radiographic evidence (see **Figure 2**), although an X-ray is less important in diagnosis than a detailed history and examination, and does not always correspond with the clinical symptoms [1].

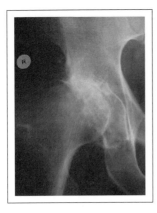

Figure 2. X-ray of an osteoarthritic hip, showing loss of joint space, sclerosis, and osteophyte formation.

Reproduced with permission from DrDoc on-line (Osteoarthritis. A review for the primary physician. www.arthritis.co.za/osteoarthritis_update.html).

Management

Evidence-based guidelines for the management of osteoarthritis, published by the Michigan Quality Improvement Consortium, are available from www.mqic.org. The guidelines are summarized in **Table 2** [10]. In addition, the Agency for Healthcare Research and Quality has published a research review entitled *Comparative Effectiveness and Safety of Analgesics for Osteoarthritis* [11]. This focuses on four key questions:

1. What is the evidence for benefits and harms of treating osteoarthritis with oral medication(s)?
2. Are there clinically important differences in the harms and benefits of oral treatments for osteoarthritis for certain demographic and clinical subgroups?
3. What is the evidence that the gastrointestinal harms of nonsteroidal anti-inflammatory drug use are reduced by co-prescribing of H_2-antagonists, misoprostol, or proton-pump inhibitors?
4. What are the benefits and safety of treating osteoarthritis with oral medications as compared with topical preparations?

The 'clinical bottom line' of this review is shown in **Table 3**. The full review is available from www.effectivehealthcare. ahrq.gov/reports/final.cfm.

Initial evaluation

Detailed history (aspirin use, pain control with over-the-counter medications, activity tolerance and limitations)

Physical examination

Assess GI risk (history of ulcer disease or GI bleeding; high-dose, chronic, or multiple NSAIDs, including aspirin; concomitant use of corticosteroids and/or warfarin; age >60 years)

Nonpharmacologic modalities

The treatment plan should include:

- education and counseling regarding weight reduction, joint protection, and energy conservation
- range of motion, aerobic, and muscle-strengthening exercises
- physical therapy and occupational therapy, if required
- assistive devices, if required
- appropriate footwear, orthotics
- self-management resources (eg, American Arthritis Foundation self-help course and book)
- complementary alternative medicine (eg, glucosamine)

Pharmacologic therapy

Non-NSAID analgesics:

- initial drug of choice: acetaminophen
- patients with organ (eg, liver, kidney) toxicity risk factors, reassess for other therapies
- tramadol, opioids, intra-articular glucocorticoids or hyaluronate, topical capsaicin

NSAID analgesics (see **Table 3**):

- patients at low cardiovascular risk who are not using aspirin:

  – no or low GI risk: use a nonselective NSAID. If GI symptoms develop, add an antacid, H_2-antagonist, or PPI

  – GI risk: use an NSAID plus PPI. Consider non-NSAID therapy

- patients at cardiovascular risk:

  – no or low GI risk: use a nonselective NSAID, plus PPI if GI risk warrants gastroprotection. Consider non-NSAID therapy

  – GI risk: a gastroprotective agent must be added if a nonselective NSAID or aspirin is prescribed. Consider non-NSAID therapy

Table 2. Summary of recommendations for the management of osteoarthritis [10]. GI: gastrointestinal; NSAID: nonsteroidal anti-inflammatory drug; PPI: proton-pump inhibitor.

Clinical bottom line	Level of confidence[a]
Acetaminophen relieves mild pain, but is inferior to NSAIDs for reducing moderate or severe inflammatory pain. Acetaminophen has fewer systemic side effects than NSAIDs	High
All non-aspirin NSAIDs work equally well for pain reduction	High
NSAIDs increase the risk of GI bleeding. The risk increases with higher doses and with age. People aged >75 years have the highest risk	High
Celecoxib, high-dose ibuprofen, and high-dose diclofenac increase the risk of MI. Naproxen does not increase the risk of MI	Medium

Table 3. The clinical bottom line from the Agency for Healthcare Research and Quality research review on choosing nonopioid analgesics for osteoarthritis [11]. [a]High: there are consistent results from good quality studies; medium: findings are supported, but further research could change the conclusions. GI: gastrointestinal; MI: myocardial infarction; NSAID: nonsteroidal anti-inflammatory drug.

References

1. Jones A, Doherty M. ABC of rheumatology. Osteoarthritis. *BMJ* 1995;310:457–60.

2. Murray CJL, Lopez AD. *The Global Burden of Disease*. Geneva: World Health Organization, 1997.

3. Arden N, Nevitt MC. Osteoarthritis: epidemiology. *Best Pract Res Clin Rheumatol* 2006;20:3–25.

4. Lawrence RC, Hochberg MC, Kelsey JL, et al. Estimates of the prevalence of selected arthritic and musculoskeletal diseases in the United States. *J Rheumatol* 1989;16:427–41.

5. Dieppe P. Osteoarthritis. A review. *J Royal Coll Phys London* 1990;24:262–7.

6. Felson DT. Epidemiology of hip and knee osteoarthritis. *Epidemiol Rev* 1988;10:1–28.

7. Steigelfest, E. Osteoarthritis. *eMedicine*, 2005. Available from: www.emedicine.com/med/topic1682.htm. Accessed July 30, 2007.

8. Rottenstein K. Public Health Agency of Canada. *Monograph Series on Aging-related Diseases IX. Osteoarthritis*. Available from: www.phac-aspc.gc.ca. Accessed July 30, 2007.

9. Simon LS, Lipman AG, Jacox AK, et al. *Pain in Osteoarthritis, Rheumatoid Arthritis, and Juvenile Chronic Arthritis*. Glenview, IL: American Pain Society, 2002.

10. Michigan Quality Improvement Consortium. *Medical Management of Adults with Osteoarthritis,* 2005. Available from www.mqic.org. Accessed July 30, 2007.

11. Chou R, Helfand M, Peterson K, et al. *Comparative Effectiveness and Safety of Analgesics for Osteoarthritis. Comparative Effectiveness Review No. 4*. Rockville, MD: Agency for Healthcare Research and Quality, 2006. Available from: www.effectivehealthcare.ahrq.gov/reports/final.cfm. Accessed July 30, 2007.

6 • Ischemic pain syndromes

Angina pectoris

Angina pectoris describes the pain or discomfort that occurs when myocardial oxygen demand exceeds supply [1,2].

> "In affluent societies, coronary artery disease causes severe disability and more death than any other disease, including cancer" [3].

Epidemiology

Recently, the Centers for Disease and Control and Prevention has collated self-reported data from the 2005 Behavioral Risk Factor Surveillance System (356,112 respondents) to give an overview of heart disease in the USA [4]. Age, gender, geographic, racial/ethnic, and educational data were all assessed:

- Men had a significantly higher prevalence of angina/ congestive heart disease (CHD) history than women (5.5% vs 3.4%).
- The prevalence of a history of angina/CHD increased among successive age groups (18–44 years, 1.1%; 45–64 years, 5.4%; ≥65 years, 13.1%) and decreased with higher education.
- American Indians/Alaska Natives and multiracial persons had substantially higher prevalences of a history of angina/CHD than non-Hispanic whites (7.2% vs 4.2%). The prevalence among whites and blacks was similar.

- Puerto Rico (8.5%) and West Virginia (7.3%) had the highest prevalence of angina/CHD history; Colorado (2.8%) and the US Virgin Islands (2.2%) had the lowest prevalence.

Risk factors
Modifiable risk factors include [5]:

- smoking (approximately doubles risk)
- hypertension (systolic blood pressure >180 mm Hg doubles risk)
- hyperlipidemia
- thrombogenic factors (eg, elevated plasma fibrinogen level)
- obesity
- glucose intolerance or diabetes
- sedentary lifestyle
- cocaine use

Pathogenesis
Coronary artery disease is usually due to atheromatous narrowing and subsequent vessel occlusion [3]. When a plaque produces a >50% diameter stenosis, reduced blood flow during exertion may lead to angina. Acute coronary events (see later) arise when thrombus formation follows disruption of a plaque.

Pain mechanisms in angina and myocardial infarction [2]
1. Ischemic episodes excite chemosensitive and mechanoreceptive receptors in the heart.
2. This leads to the release of a variety of chemicals, including adenosine and bradykinin, which excite nociceptors along the visceral afferent pathway.
3. Visceral afferent fibers from the heart enter the upper thoracic spinal cord (Th1–Th4) and synapse on cells of origin of ascending pathways.
4. Excitation of spinothalamic tract cells in the upper thoracic and lower cervical segments contributes to the anginal pain experienced in the chest and arm.
5. The vagal nerve is the 10th cranial nerve, which terminates in the nucleus tractus solitarii in the brainstem.

Crushing retrosternal chest pain
Usually lasts longer than 10 minutes
Unrelieved by rest or sublingual nitroglycerin
Radiates to right or left arm, neck, jaw, back, shoulders, or abdomen
May be associated with dyspnea, sweating, nausea, or vomiting
Pain may be absent in 20% of patients, mostly elderly or diabetics ('silent infarction')

Table 1. Characteristics of pain in myocardial infarction.

Descending impulses from here may excite upper cervical spinothalamic tract cells. This may contribute to the anginal pain experienced in the neck and jaw.

6. The spinothalamic tract activates hypothalamic, reticular, and thalamic loci and the prefrontal cortex, but not the cortical sensory areas (SI and SII) behind the central sulcus. This differentiates central visceral pain perception from somatic pain perception.

The pain mechanisms in myocardial infarction (MI) are similar to those of angina, in that a number of substances (eg, potassium, lactate, adenosine, bradykinin, and prostaglandins) are released from the damaged tissue. These then sensitize and excite the sensory nerve endings in the heart. Also, as in angina, a number of factors relating to the pain pathways contribute to difficulties in localization; there is no cortical area for the exact localization of cardiac pain. Pain is frequently radiated to the neck, arms, or back (see **Table 1**).

Clinical presentation [1,6,7]

Most patients complain of substernal chest pain. This is usually dull and associated with tightness, but is sometimes a stabbing pain. The pain or discomfort commonly radiates to the neck, jaw, shoulders, or arms, and lasts <10 minutes.

- In *stable* (chronic) angina, pain occurs on exertion (eg, climbing stairs) or may be precipitated by cold or emotional excitement.
- In *unstable* angina, pain is of new onset and occurs at rest or with minimal exertion.

Myocardial infarction
Q-wave MI on ECG
Non-Q-wave MI (enzyme release + no appearance of Q-wave on ECG)

Angina pectoris
Unstable angina pectoris
Stress-induced angina pectoris
Rest angina pectoris
Decubitus angina pectoris
Postprandial angina pectoris
Walk-through angina pectoris
Spasm angina pectoris
Silent myocardial ischemia

MI irreversibly damages the heart muscle, while angina pectoris occurs due to reversible myocardial ischemia. When myocardial ischemia is not followed by pain or discomfort it is called 'silent ischemia'. Syndrome X pain and bruise pain constitute pain syndromes similar to angina pectoris, but with no conclusive evidence of myocardial ischemia MI.

Table 2. Classification of myocardial infarction (MI) and angina pectoris in clinical states. ECG: electrocardiogram.

Reproduced with permission from Churchill Livingstone (Sylven C, Eriksson BE. Thorax. In: McMahon SB, Koltzenburg M, Editors. *Wall and Melzack's Textbook of Pain.* Churchill Livingstone, 2006:737–52).

The classification of MI and angina pectoris is shown in **Table 2**.

> "All patients [with chest pain] should be referred to a cardiologist to clarify the diagnosis, optimize drug treatment, and assess the need and suitability for revascularization" [3].

Diagnosis

Most patients can be diagnosed as having definite or possible angina on the history alone [3].

- The most widely used test in evaluating angina is a 'stress test', in which a positive result shows poor exercise capacity and ischemic changes observed following electrocardiography.
- Echocardiography may be helpful in diagnosis, eg, in evaluating left ventricular function in patients with

angina pectoris. In MI (see later), echocardiography can identify wall motion abnormalities or identify mural thrombus or mitral regurgitation, both of which may occur following an MI.

Management

Table 3 sets out the main components of a treatment plan, with recommendations primarily based on those of the American College of Cardiology/American Heart Association [5]. The treatment options set out in **Table 3** should be guided by specialist advice.

Nitrates represent the mainstay of pain relief: drugs such as nitroglycerin bring about venodilatation and relaxation of vascular smooth muscle; the decreased venous return from venodilatation decreases diastolic ventricular wall tension (preload) and thus reduces mechanical activity (and myocardial oxygen consumption) during systole [4].

Patients may be referred to a cardiologist for consideration of revascularization. Patients who should be referred include those with valvular disorders that require repair, angina that is refractory to maximal medical therapy, or comorbidities that complicate therapy [5].

Myocardial infarction

MI is characterized by necrosis resulting from an insufficient supply of oxygenated blood to an area of the heart [6,8]. It is usually divided into two categories:

- *Non-ST-segment elevation* (non-Q-wave) – the area of ischemic necrosis is limited to the inner one-third to half of the myocardial wall.
- *ST-segment elevation* (Q-wave) – the area of ischemic necrosis penetrates the full thickness of the ventricular wall.

Detailed guidelines for the diagnosis and management of MI have been published by the American College of Cardiology/

Nonpharmacologic therapy
Aggressive modification of preventable risk factors (eg, weight reduction, exercise programs, correction of lipid abnormalities, hypertension, smoking cessation)
Correction of other aggravating factors (eg, anemia, thyrotoxicosis)
Acute pharmacotherapy
Nitrates (eg, sublingual nitroglycerin or nitroglycerin spray for the immediate relief of angina)
Beta-blockers to reduce heart rate and blood pressure
Calcium-channel blockers
Aspirin (or clopidogrel when aspirin is contraindicated)
Heparin may be advised in unstable angina
Chronic pharmacotherapy
This normally includes the above, plus lipid-lowering drugs in patients with coronary heart disease or hyperlipidemia refractory to diet and exercise
Coronary artery bypass grafting
Coronary artery bypass grafting may be offered where there is significant two-vessel or three-vessel disease, or significant left main coronary disease (eg, causing substantial ischemia and/or handicap)
For refractory angina, the following is an option:
Spinal cord stimulation

Table 3. The main components in the management of chronic stable angina [1,5,6,9,10].

American Heart Association [11], and can be found at www.guideline.gov. Key recommendations include:

• Anyone with a suspected MI should be treated as an emergency, and transported to hospital by ambulance.
• Patients should receive oxygen 1–2 L/min by nasal prongs or 4–6 L/min by Venturi mask.
• Pain relief is a major element in the early management of MI.

Pain management should be directed towards acute relief of the symptoms of MI and necrosis, and towards relief of anxiety and apprehension, which can increase pain perception. Morphine sulfate is the analgesic of choice, except in patients with documented morphine sensitivity. Give 2–4 mg IV, repeated at 5- to 15-minute intervals. Anxiety reduction secondary to morphine administration reduces the patient's restlessness and the activity of the autonomic nervous system, with a consequent reduction in the heart's metabolic demands. Morphine administration is also beneficial in patients with pulmonary edema [11].

The side effects of morphine administration, such as hypotension, can be minimized by keeping the patient supine and elevating the lower extremities if blood pressure falls to <100 mm Hg systolic. Respiratory depression is relatively uncommon. However, respiration should be monitored, and the μ-opioid receptor antagonist naloxone, 0.1–0.2 mg IV, can be given initially if indicated, and repeated after 15 minutes if necessary [11].

Intermittent claudication

Claudication is derived from the Latin word '*claudicatio*', meaning 'to limp'. It is a descriptive term for exercise-induced leg pain that is relieved by rest [12]. Intermittent claudication affects >5 million people in the USA [13]. It is associated with an increased risk of mortality, nonfatal cardiovascular disease (MI, congestive heart failure, and cerebrovascular disease), and impaired lower extremity function [14].

Intermittent claudication can be caused by any occlusive lesion in the arterial supply of the leg muscles that interferes sufficiently with blood flow to cause ischemic pain with exercise. However, at least in the Western world, by far the most common cause is atherosclerosis [15].

Risk factor	Comment
Cigarette smoking	The most potent risk factor, with a dose-related positive correlation
	Relative risk is 1.75 at 11–20 cigarettes per day and 2.11 at >20 cigarettes per day
Age	Risk increases with age; at least 10% of people aged >70 years are affected
Diabetes	Up to 20% of patients with peripheral arterial disease have diabetes, which is often undiagnosed at the time of presentation
	Diabetes raises the risk of peripheral arterial disease by 2- to 3-fold, in turn increasing the risk of claudication
Hypertension	Hypertension strongly contributes to risk, and also to the risk of comorbid cardiac disease and mortality
Hypercholesterolemia	Significantly contributes to risk
Physical inactivity	Significantly contributes to risk
Increasing body mass	Significantly contributes to risk

Table 4. Risk factors for intermittent claudication [11,15,18].

By far the most common cause of intermittent claudication is atherosclerosis. The most potent risk factor for claudication is cigarette smoking (see **Table 4**).

Pathogenesis

Claudication develops in muscle that is distal to a main artery that has become either completely or partially obstructed, usually by atherosclerosis. This obstruction means that an exercising muscle cannot obtain enough blood to meet its increased metabolic demands. Pain occurs because the flow of blood is insufficient to remove metabolic waste products [12,16,17].

Collateral vessels form around the arterial obstruction so that the blood flow is adequate at rest; however, the total resistance of the collateral vessels is always greater than that of the major artery they are replacing, and blood flow therefore becomes inadequate to meet the increased demands of exercise [18].

Diagnosis

Clinical presentation

The pain of intermittent claudication has three characteristics [19]:

- it is a cramping pain in the calves, brought on by exertion
- it is relieved by rest
- it is 'reproducible'; that is, it almost always occurs after having walked the same distance – although it may occur earlier if the patient walks uphill or more quickly

> Claudication can be diagnosed with relative certainty based on the history and physical examination [20].

Physical examination

Diagnosis is usually based on the medical history and physical examination [20]. On examination, there is likely to be evidence of peripheral arterial occlusive disease, such as absent or decreased peripheral pulses, decreased skin temperature, shiny, hairless skin over the lower extremities, dystrophic toenails, pallor and increased pain on elevation of the extremity, and rubor when the limb is dependent. It is important that the examination and history include screening for major risk factors (eg, hypertension, diabetes).

Investigations

Investigations such as arteriography or magnetic resonance angiography are rarely required for the initial diagnosis of intermittent claudication [20]. Assessment of Doppler segmental pressure, with calculation of the ankle–brachial index, may provide helpful information about the degree of suspected arterial obstruction [12]. Doppler segmental pressures are obtained by placing blood pressure cuffs around the arm and at the proximal thigh, distal thigh, proximal calf, and ankle of the affected leg. The ankle–brachial index constitutes a sensitive means of detecting reduced blood flow in the lower limb. **Table 5** shows the differential diagnosis.

Diagnosis	Description
Venous claudication	Pain in the entire leg, but worse in the calf
	Pain occurs after walking and subsides slowly (quicker with elevation)
	The patient may have a history of iliofemoral deep vein thrombosis, and signs of venous compression or edema
Symptomatic Baker's cyst	Occurs with exercise, but is also present at rest
	The pain is not intermittent
Tightness and pain in the calf in athletes (chronic compartment syndrome)	Occurs mainly in heavily muscled athletes
	Follows vigorous exercise and does not subside quickly with rest
Nerve root compression	Pain radiates down the leg
	Often present at rest
Spinal stenosis (neurogenic claudication)	Often bilateral
	Worse with standing and extending spine; relieved by lumbar spine flexion

Table 5. Differential diagnosis of intermittent claudication [15].

Management

Table 6 lists the recommended components of best medical treatment for intermittent claudication.

Comprehensive guidelines for the diagnosis and management of peripheral arterial disease have been published by the TransAtlantic Inter-Society Consensus, and are available at www.tasc-pad.org.

Sickle cell disease

Sickle cell disease is a disorder of hemoglobin synthesis, inherited as an autosomal recessive gene. Pain is the most frequent problem for patients with sickle cell disease.

Treatment	Comment
Risk factor modification	Eg, smoking cessation, control of diabetes, hypertension, and lipids, diabetic foot care
Exercise rehabilitation	Supervised exercise training should be performed for a minimum of 30–45 minutes, in sessions performed at least 3 times/week for a minimum of 3 months
Antiplatelet therapy	Eg, aspirin, clopidogrel
Claudication therapies	A therapeutic trial of cilostazol should be considered in all patients with lifestyle-limiting claudication (in the absence of heart failure)
	Pentoxifylline may be considered as a second-line alternative to cilostazol
Endovascular procedures	Indicated for individuals with a vocational or lifestyle-limiting claudication, when clinical features suggest a reasonable likelihood of symptomatic improvement with endovascular intervention and:
	• there has been an inadequate response to exercise or pharmacologic therapy; and/or
	• there is a very favorable risk–benefit ratio
Surgical interventions	Indicated for individuals who:
	• have a significant functional disability that is vocational or lifestyle limiting
	• are unresponsive to exercise or pharmacotherapy
	• have a reasonable likelihood of symptomatic improvement

Table 6. American College of Cardiology/American Heart Association recommendations for the treatment of intermittent claudication [21]. BID: twice daily; PO: by mouth; TID: three times daily.

Epidemiology

Sickle cell disease was first described in Grenada in 1910; it occurs almost exclusively in people of African descent. It is widespread in Africa, the Middle East, Mediterranean countries, and India, and has been carried, by population movement, to the Caribbean, North America, and Europe [22].

- Sickle cell disease is most common in African Americans, with 1 in 500 African Americans born with the disease [23].
- Over 70,000 Americans currently have sickle cell disease [23].

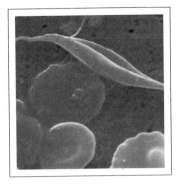

Figure 1. Normal (round), serrated, and sickle-shaped red blood cells.

Reproduced with permission from the Wellcome Trust (EM Unit, Royal Free Hospital School of Medicine/Wellcome Photo Library).

- Sickle cell disease substantially reduces life expectancy; the median life expectancies are 42 and 48 years for affected men and women, respectively [24].
- Infection is the most common cause of death in children aged 1–3 years, while stroke and trauma are the most common causes in patients aged >10 years [25].

Pathogenesis

Sickle cell disease results from an amino acid substitution (valine for glutamate) in position 6 of the beta globin chain for hemoglobin, leading to the production of hemoglobin S. When exposed to lower oxygen tension, hemoglobin S undergoes aggregation and polymerization in the red cells, which become deformed and commonly sickle-shaped (see **Figure 1**) [26].

The clinical problems (eg, painful crises) encountered in sickle cell disease result from vaso-occlusion, as the sickle-shaped erythrocyte is rigid, deforms poorly, and can adhere to the vascular endothelium [27]. Ischemia leads to pain and organ damage (see **Figure 2**).

Clinical presentation

The most common symptom of sickle cell disease is pain. Severe pain can occur in patients as young as 6 months, and may continue throughout the patient's life [28]. Patients can also experience other health problems, such as frequent infections, anemia, and skin ulcers (see **Figure 3**) [23].

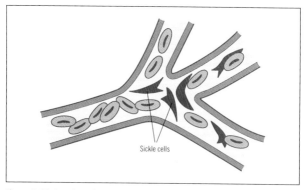

Figure 2. Obstruction of blood vessels by sickle cells.

Reproduced with permission from the Ohio Sickle Cell & Health Association (*Effects of Sickle Cell Disease*. Available from: www.ohiosicklecell.org/effects.html).

Anemia

Anemia does not invariably occur in sickle cell disease, but hemoglobin levels are usually between 7 and 10 g/dL, and the blood picture shows anisocytosis, sickle cells, and a raised reticulocyte count due to accelerated erythropoiesis. The anemia can be severe, and blood transfusions may be necessary [29].

Infection

Sickle cell patients are prone to infections, including serious and life-threatening infections such as septicemia, meningococcal meningitis, and osteomyelitis [29].

Pain

- Pain is the most frequent problem for people with sickle cell disease, and it profoundly affects quality of life and functioning in work, school, social life, and relationships.
- Pain can be precipitated by stimuli such as dehydration, fatigue, cold weather, an infection, and exercising too hard [23], but not all painful episodes have a clear precipitant.
- Pain has been reported to occur on up to 30% of days, with a loss of 10% of schooldays for children [30].

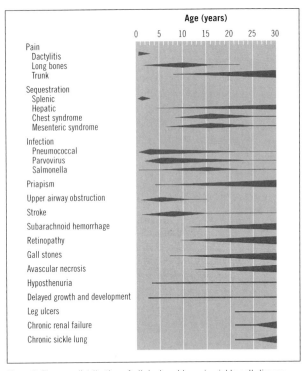

Figure 3. The age distribution of clinical problems in sickle cell disease.

Reproduced with permission from *BMJ* Journals (Davies SC, Oni L. Management of patients with sickle cell disease. *BMJ* 1997;315:656–60).

- Painful and symmetric swelling of the hands and feet (hand–foot syndrome) caused by infarctions of the small bones may be the first manifestation of the disease. It is usually seen in children aged <4 years, and is very uncommon after 7 years. Osteonecrosis comes later (see **Figure 4**); infarction is the cause [27].

> Pain is the most frequent problem for people with sickle cell disease, and profoundly affects quality of life and functioning in work, school, social life, and relationships.

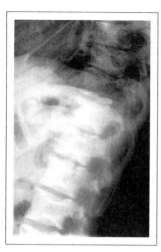

Figure 4. Bony changes in sickle cell disease. Osteonecrosis and collapse of multiple thoracic vertebral end plates in a 29-year-old woman with sickle cell disease and recurrent bone pain.

Reproduced with permission from Michael L. Richardson, MD, University of Washington Department of Radiology (*Musculoskeletal Manifestations of Sickle Cell Disease.* Available from: http://uwmsk.org/resident projects/sicklecell.html.)

Patients' self-reports should be the main source of pain assessment, with the exception of infants or patients with cognitive dysfunction, for whom behavioral observations are the primary source of assessment
For rapid pain assessment during an acute event, physicians should select a simple measurement of pain intensity and reassess the patient frequently for response to treatment
Patients should have a comprehensive clinical assessment of their pain every year, and more often if pain is more frequent
When physicians observe a disparity between a patient's verbal self-report of their pain and their ability to function, further assessment should address the reason for the disparity

Table 7. Pain assessment in sickle cell disease [28].

Assessment

Table 7 summarizes the recommendations of the American Pain Society for pain assessment in sickle cell disease [28]. Assessment is best performed between acute episodes.

Management

Sickle cell disease is a complex, heterogeneous, and chronic disorder. **Table 8** briefly summarizes the American Pain Society recommendations for the treatment of pain in sickle cell disease.

Pain management should be aggressive to ease pain and enable patients to attain maximal functional ability
Analgesics are the foundation of pain management, their use should be tailored to each patient
Nonsteroidal anti-inflammatory drugs should be prescribed for mild pain unless contraindicated; if ineffective, an opioid should be added
Opioid tolerance and physical dependence should not be confused with psychological dependence
Sedatives and anxiolytics should not be used alone to manage pain
Severe pain should be considered a medical emergency, and timely and aggressive management should be provided until the pain becomes tolerable
Equianalgesic doses of oral opioids should be provided for home use where necessary

Table 8. Treatment of pain in sickle cell disease [28].

As in other painful disorders – and especially so in sickle cell disease – pain management needs to be part of a comprehensive treatment plan that should, wherever possible, include patient education, family support, and cognitive behavioral therapy [31].

References

1. Solomon AJ, Gersh BJ. Management of chronic stable angina: medical therapy, percutaneous transluminal coronary angioplasty, and coronary artery bypass graft surgery. Lessons from the randomized trials. *Ann Intern Med* 1998;128:216–23.

2. Foreman RD. Mechanisms of cardiac pain. *Annu Rev Physiol* 1999;61:143–67.

3. Grech ED. Pathophysiology and investigation of coronary artery disease. *BMJ* 2003;326:1027–30.

4. Centers for Disease Control and Prevention (CDC). Prevalence of heart disease – United States, 2005. *MMWR Morb Mortal Wkly Rep* 2007;56:113–18.

5. Gibbons RJ, Abrams J, Chatterjee K, et al. for the American College of Cardiology; American Heart Association Task Force on practice guidelines (Committee on the Management of Patients With Chronic Stable Angina). ACC/AHA 2002 guideline update for the management of patients with chronic stable angina – summary article: a report of the American College of Cardiology/American Heart Association Task Force on practice guidelines (Committee on the Management of Patients With Chronic Stable Angina). *J Am Coll Cardiol* 2003;41:159–68.

6. Ferri FF, Editor. *Ferri's Clinical Advisor*. St Louis: Mosby, 2000.

7. Green CB, Harris IS, Lin GA, et al., Editors. *The Washington Manual of Medical Therapeutics*, 31st edn. Philadelphia: Lippincott Williams & Wilkins, 2004.

8. Grech ED, Ramsdale DR. Acute coronary syndrome: unstable angina and non-ST segment elevation myocardial infarction. *BMJ* 2003;326:1259–61.

9. Simpson BA, Meyerson BA, Linderoth B. Spinal cord and brain stimulation. In: McMahon SB, Koltzenburg M, Editors. *Wall and Melzack's Textbook of Pain*. London: Churchill Livingstone, 2006:563–82.

10. Hautvast RW, DeJongste MJ, Staal MJ, et al. Spinal cord stimulation in chronic intractable angina pectoris: a randomized, controlled efficacy study. *Am Heart J* 1998;136:1114–20.

11. Antman EM, Anbe DT, Armstrong PW, et al. ACC/AHA guidelines for the management of patients with ST-elevation myocardial infarction; a report of the American College of Cardiology/American Heart Association Task Force on Practice Guidelines (Committee to Revise the 1999 Guidelines for the Management of patients with acute myocardial infarction). *J Am Coll Cardiol* 2004;44:E1–E211.

12. Santilli JD, Rodnick JE, Santilli SM. Claudication: diagnosis and treatment. *Am Fam Physician* 1996;53:1245–53.

13. Selvin E, Erlinger TP. Prevalence of and risk factors for peripheral arterial disease in the United States: results from the National Health and Nutrition Examination Survey, 1999–2000. *Circulation* 2004;110:738–43.

14. Murabito JM, Evans JC, D'Agostino RB, et al. Temporal trends in the incidence of intermittent claudication from 1950 to 1999. *Am J Epidemiol* 2005;162:430–7.

15. Norgren L, Hiatt WR, Dormandy JA, et al. for the TASC II Working Group. Inter-society consensus for the management of peripheral arterial disease (TASC II). *Eur J Vasc Endovasc Surg* 2007;33:S1–70.

16. Hiatt WR, Stoll S, Nies AS. Effect of beta-adrenergic blockers on the peripheral circulation in patients with peripheral vascular disease. *Circulation* 1985;72:1226–31.

17. Gardner AW. Dissipation of claudication pain after walking: implications for endurance training. *Med Sci Sports Exerc* 1993;25:904–10.

18. Bowlin SJ, Medalie JH, Flocke SA, et al. Epidemiology of intermittent claudication in middle-aged men. *Am J Epidemiol* 1994;140:418–30.

19. Heart Canada. *Intermittent Claudication*. Available from: www.heartcanada.com/claudication.php. Accessed July 30, 2007.

20. Carman TL, Fernandez BB Jr. A primary care approach to the patient with claudication. *Am Fam Physician* 2000;61:1027–32,1034.

21. Writing Committee to Develop Guidelines for the Management of Patients With Peripheral Arterial Disease. ACC/AHA 2005 Guidelines for the Management of Patients With Peripheral Arterial Disease (Lower Extremity, Renal, Mesenteric, and Abdominal Aortic): Executive Summary. *J Am Coll Cardiol* 2006;47:1239–312.

22. Davies SC, Oni L. Management of patients with sickle cell disease. *BMJ* 1997;315:656–60.

23. Department of Pain Medicine and Palliative Care, Beth Israel Medical Center. *Sickle Cell Pain*. Available from: www.StopPain.org. Accessed July 30, 2007.

24. Platt OS, Brambilla DJ, Rosse WF, et al. Mortality in sickle cell disease – life expectancy and risk factors for early death. *N Engl J Med* 1994;330:1639–44.

25. Leikin SL, Gallagher D, Kinney TR, et al. Mortality in children and adolescents with sickle cell disease. *Pediatrics* 1989;84:500–8.

26. Bunn HF. Pathogenesis and treatment of sickle cell disease. *N Engl J Med* 1997;337:762–9.

27. Frenette PS. Sickle cell vaso-occlusion: multistep and multicellular paradigm. *Curr Opin Hematol* 2002;9:101–6.

28. American Pain Society. *Guideline for the Management of Acute and Chronic Pain in Sickle-Cell Disease*. Available from: www.ampainsoc.org. Accessed July 30, 2007.

29. Sickle Cell Society. *Information for Health Professionals*. Available from: www.sicklecellsociety.org. Accessed July 30, 2007.

30. Shapiro BS, Dinges DF, Orne EC, et al. Home management of sickle cell-related pain in children and adolescents: natural history and impact on school attendance. *Pain* 1995;61:139–44.

31. Preboth M. Management of pain in sickle cell disease. *Am Fam Physician* 2000;61:1549–50.

7 • Visceral pain syndromes

Painful visceral disorders are commonly experienced, with many people suffering from irritable bowel syndrome (IBS), dysmenorrhea, and/or chronic pelvic pain (CPP). Visceral pain syndromes are often chronic, recurring, and, in many cases, fairly resistant to treatment.

Visceral pain

Visceral pain is a frequent reason for gastroenterological referrals. It is diffuse and can be difficult to localize. As several viscera can converge onto the same spinal segment, patterns of referred sensations can overlap considerably, causing problems with differential diagnosis.

Visceral pain involves sensitization processes similar to those in somatic pain, and may involve the activation of previously silent nociceptors (see **Chapter 1**). This can lead to a chronic hyperalgesic state [1].

Visceral pain affects basic physiological functions such as eating, defecation, and urination. It is also often associated with vegetative symptoms such as nausea, vomiting, dizziness, and anxiety. A major problem with the treatment of visceral pain is that adverse reactions to analgesics can include disturbed visceral function, such as nausea, constipation, gastric irritation, ulceration, and urinary retention. This must be taken into account when therapy is considered [2].

Irritable bowel syndrome

IBS is typically characterized by abdominal pain, altered bowel function (eg, increased bowel frequency, constipation), bloating, abdominal distension, the sensation of incomplete evacuation, and the increased passage of mucus. No single hypothesis explains all of these clinical features.

> "[IBS] is probably the most common disorder encountered by gastroenterologists in the industrialized world and the most common functional bowel disorder seen in primary care" [3].

Epidemiology

The American Gastroenterological Association's (AGA) *Technical Review on Irritable Bowel Syndrome* summarizes the epidemiologic features of this common disorder [4]. In brief:

- IBS is more prevalent in women than in men.
- The first presentation of patients to a physician is generally between the ages of 30 and 50 years.
- The prevalence of IBS appears to be similar in whites and African Americans, but may be lower in people of Hispanic origin.

Furthermore, many people with IBS symptoms do not seek medical attention. For example, a survey by Hungin et al., based on >5,000 screening interviews, found that clinicians see only a minority of sufferers [5]. In their survey, there was a total IBS prevalence of 14.1%. Only 3.3% of this was accounted for by medically diagnosed patients, with 10.8% made up of people who were undiagnosed, but who met IBS criteria (Manning, Rome I, or Rome II). They concluded that 76.6% of IBS sufferers are undiagnosed.

Pathogenesis

No clear cause of IBS has been identified. The currently favored model involves both central and end-organ components – that

Pain eased after bowel movement
Looser stools at onset of pain
More frequent bowel movements at onset of pain
Abdominal distension (bloating)
Mucus in stools
Feeling of incomplete emptying

Table 1. Symptoms that are more likely to be found in irritable bowel syndrome than in organic abdominal disease [8].

is, a combination of psychological factors (eg, stress, affective disorder) and dysfunction of the gut (eg, disorders of motility, visceral hypersensitivity) [4]. For example:

- Gastroenteritis (any form) may predispose patients to the development of IBS [4].
- Symptoms of anxiety or depression, or other stress symptoms, have been noted in 40–60% of patients [3,6].
- Innovative use of positron emission tomography and functional magnetic resonance imaging scans has demonstrated altered brain activity and regional blood flow in IBS patients [7].

Clinical presentation

There are no agreed diagnostic criteria for IBS, but the Manning criteria list features that are more likely to be due to IBS than organic disease (see **Table 1**) [8]; these have been well validated [3]. Other criteria in common use are the Rome criteria. The more recent Rome III criteria are considered less restrictive than the Rome II criteria, and may more closely reflect the socioeconomic burden of IBS [9,10].

Characteristics of abdominal discomfort

- The abdominal pain or discomfort may take the form of bloating, a feeling of distension, or of sharp, stabbing, or crampy pain.
- Some patients describe a 'squeezing' sensation.
- There is considerable variability in the frequency and intensity of symptoms. Some patients are temporarily incapacitated by their symptoms.

Red flags
Age >50 years
GI bleeding
Anemia
Weight loss
Severe diarrhea
Fever
Family history of colorectal cancer, inflammatory bowel disease, or celiac disease
Vomiting
Recent travel to areas known for enteric pathogens

Table 2. Red flags in diagnosis of irritable bowel syndrome. GI: gastrointestinal.

Reproduced with permission from Medical Economics (Horwitz BL, Lembo AJ, Whitehead WE. Managing irritable bowel syndrome. *Patient Care* 2003;2:18–34).

- Consider IBS when the discomfort is exacerbated by eating or stress, associated with a change in the frequency or consistency of the stool, and/or relieved by defecation [4].

Differential diagnosis

The main differentials are inflammatory bowel disease, colorectal polyps or cancers, malabsorption (lactose intolerance or celiac disease), infectious diarrhea, and thyroid dysfunction. Physicians should be alert for 'red flag' or 'alarm feature' signs, which indicate that a diagnosis other than IBS must be excluded (see **Table 2**) [7].

Management

The AGA has summarized management strategies that are useful in IBS (see **Table 3**) [4,9]. Points to note are:

- A common treatment strategy is to focus on the symptom(s) that the patient finds most troublesome, eg, pain, diarrhea, emotional distress.
- Antispasmodic (anticholinergic) medication (eg, dicyclomine, mebeverine) should be considered for the treatment of pain and bloating, particularly when the symptoms are exacerbated by meals. Use on an as-needed basis, up to three times a day.

Management	Comment
Consider red flags	See **Table 2**
Reassurance and education	Reassurance should follow once the physician has elicited the patient's worries and concerns, and after an adequate and generally conservative diagnostic examination
Dietary modification	The type of food does not generally contribute to symptoms, although certain foods may aggravate symptoms in some individuals
	Care should be taken to avoid an unnecessarily restrictive diet
	The value of fiber in the relief of IBS-related diarrhea is controversial, and fiber is not helpful for pain
Symptom monitoring	It may be useful for the patient to keep a symptom diary for 2–3 weeks
Symptom-targeted pharmacotherapy	Antispasmodic (anticholinergic) medications for pain and bloating
	Low-dose TCAs (eg, 10–50 mg/day) for more constant and/or disabling pain
	Increased dietary fiber (25 g/day) or osmotic laxatives for constipation
	Loperamide for diarrhea
	5-HT$_3$ antagonists – see main text
Complementary/ alternative therapies	Efficacy has not been established in randomized controlled trials
Psychological treatment	Consider when symptoms are moderate to severe, when patients are refractory to medical treatment, or when stress or psychological factors are contributing to symptom exacerbation
	No studies indicate that one psychological intervention technique is superior to another
Centrally targeted (psychotropic) medications	Antidepressants (eg, TCAs, SSRIs) and anxiolytic agents (eg, benzodiazepines) are commonly prescribed for IBS
	Full doses of TCAs (eg, 100–150 mg/day) may be effective when low doses are not

Table 3. Treatment strategies in irritable bowel syndrome. Recommendations from the American Gastroenterological Association [4,9]. 5-HT$_3$: 5-hydroxytryptamine-3; IBS: irritable bowel syndrome; SSRI: selective serotonin reuptake inhibitor; TCA: tricyclic antidepressant.

Earlier age at menarche
Nulliparity
Long menstrual periods/heavier menstrual flow
Smoking
No oral contraceptive use
Obesity
Alcohol consumption
Attempting to lose weight
Depression

Table 4. Possible risk factors for dysmenorrhea [11–13].

- Low-dose tricyclic antidepressants may be considered when the pain is more constant and/or disabling.
- Some newer strategies involve drugs that modify the effects of 5-hydroxytryptamine (5-HT) in the gut. Alosetron hydrochloride, a selective 5-HT$_3$ antagonist, is effective in relieving pain, and normalizing bowel frequency, and reducing urgency in female patients with diarrhea-predominant IBS. Alosetron is approved by the Food and Drug Administration under restrictive guidelines.

Dysmenorrhea

Dysmenorrhea may be primary (with no identifiable underlying disease) or secondary, most commonly to endometriosis. Other causes include fibromas and pelvic inflammatory disease [10].

There are no widely agreed risk factors for primary dysmenorrhea. Risk factors that have been identified in some studies – although not in all – are listed in **Table 4** [11–13].

- *Primary* dysmenorrhea is defined as menstrual pain not associated with macroscopic pelvic pathology. It occurs in the first few years after menarche and affects approximately 50% of postpubescent females [11].

- *Secondary* dysmenorrhea is defined as menstrual pain resulting from anatomic and/or macroscopic pelvic pathology. It is most often seen in women aged 30–45 years [11].

Epidemiology

- Approximately 50% of menstruating women are affected by dysmenorrhea, although some studies indicate that up to 90% of women experience dysmenorrhea at some point in their lives [14]. It is the most common gynecological problem in menstruating women.
- Some 10% of affected women have severe symptoms, with incapacity for 1–3 days [15].
- Onset is usually 6–12 months after menarche [16].
- Dysmenorrhea is associated with activity restriction and school or work absence in 10–45% of sufferers [16].
- In 1984, it was calculated that dysmenorrhea accounted for 600 million lost work hours and $2 billion in lost productivity per year [17].

Etiology

The etiology of dysmenorrhea is not fully established, but there is evidence to support a central role for uterine prostaglandins, particularly prostaglandin $F_{2\alpha}$ [13].

- During endometrial sloughing, the disintegrating endometrial cells release prostaglandin $F_{2\alpha}$ as menstruation begins.
- Prostaglandin $F_{2\alpha}$ stimulates myometrial contractions, ischemia, and sensitization of sensory nerve endings.
- Women who have more severe dysmenorrhea have higher levels of prostaglandin $F_{2\alpha}$ in their menstrual fluid.
- Many studies have documented the efficacy of nonsteroidal anti-inflammatory drugs (NSAIDs), which act through cyclooxygenase inhibition [11].

> "A focused history and physical examination are usually sufficient to make the diagnosis of primary dysmenorrhea" [13].

Adenomyosis
Pelvic inflammatory disease
Cervical stenosis and polyps
Fibroids (intracavitary or intramural; including leiomyofibromas)
Intrauterine contraceptive device
Infection
Endometriosis
Inflammation and scarring (eg, adhesions)
Functional ovarian cysts
Benign or malignant tumors of the uterus, ovary, bowel, bladder, or other site
Inflammatory bowel disease

Table 5. Possible causes of secondary dysmenorrhea.

Reproduced with permission from the American Academy of Family Physicians (Coco AS. Primary dysmenorrhea. *Am Fam Physician* 1999;60:689–96).

Clinical presentation

- The pain of dysmenorrhea is often sharp and crampy, and centered in the suprapubic area. The pain may radiate to the back of the legs or the lower back.
- Frequent accompanying symptoms include nausea, vomiting, headache, anxiety, fatigue, diarrhea, and abdominal bloating.
- In primary dysmenorrhea, a pelvic examination is usually normal.
- In secondary dysmenorrhea (see **Table 5**), dyspareunia is a common complaint; a pelvic–abdominal examination may reveal uterine or adnexal tenderness, fixed uterine retroflexion, a pelvic mass, or an enlarged, irregular uterus.

Management

NSAIDs are the most effective drug treatment, with a Cochrane review concluding that there is overwhelming evidence for the effectiveness of NSAIDs in providing pain relief from dysmenorrhea [18]. They are thought to work by inhibiting prostaglandin synthesis, thus decreasing prostaglandin levels and reducing uterine contractility. NSAIDs also seem to decrease excessive menstrual bleeding volume.

> **Box 1.** Caution: risks of NSAID use [19].
>
> When treating women with risk factors for NSAID-induced ulceration, the potential risks and benefits should be considered. Risk factors for NSAID-induced ulceration include:
>
> - Previous clinical history of gastroduodenal ulcer or ulcer complications.
> - Concomitant use of medications known to increase the likelihood of gastrointestinal GI bleeding (eg, glucocorticosteroids, low-dose aspirin, antidepressants [selective serotonin reuptake inhibitors/serotonin and norepinephrine reuptake inhibitors], anticoagulants).
> - Presence of major comorbidity (eg, cardiovascular disease, diabetes, hypertension).
> - No previous NSAID use (versus long-term NSAID use).
>
> Note that NSAID-induced GI complications (including ulceration, perforation, and the development of strictures) can appear from the esophagus to the rectum. It has been estimated that 25–40% of serious complications occur outside of the stomach and duodenum. Conventional prophylaxis with proton-pump inhibitors or H_2-receptor blockers does not affect complications in these areas [20].

There is no clear evidence supporting one NSAID over another, but ibuprofen and naproxen are widely used and recommended. Oral contraceptives can also be effective, and behavioral interventions may be of some use [16].

Chronic pelvic pain

This is an area in which terminology is not fully agreed upon, and where descriptive terms can be problematic. Here, we define CPP as a female syndrome of nonmenstrual pain of ≥3 months' duration that localizes to the anatomic pelvis, and is severe enough to cause functional disability and require medical or surgical treatment [21]. The disorder, although common, is still poorly understood.

Epidemiology

- CPP affects approximately one in seven women [22].
  Of all referrals to gynecologists, 10% are for pelvic pain.

- CPP is most common among those aged 26–30 years [14].
- The direct costs for CPP-related outpatient visits have been estimated at approximately $881.5 million per year [22].
- CPP can lead to prolonged suffering, family problems, disability, and loss of employment.
- Risk factors may include nonblack ethnicity, being married, poor mental health, and smoking [23].

Etiology

There is no single established cause of CPP. As many as 61% of women who experience the disorder never receive a specific diagnosis [24]. CPP shares the common characteristic of visceral pain in being difficult to localize. Underlying disorders can include:

- extrauterine disorders (eg, endometriosis, adhesions)
- uterine disorders (eg, adenomyosis, atypical dysmenorrhea)
- urological disorders (eg, urinary tract infection)
- musculoskeletal disorders (eg, fibromyalgia)
- GI disorders (eg, colitis [including diverticulitis], colon cancer)
- psychological disorders (eg, anxiety, depression, sexual/physical abuse)

Pain in CPP

There is no typical pattern of pain in CPP. The features can include:

- severe and steady pain
- intermittent pain
- dull aching
- sharp pains or cramping
- pressure or heaviness deep within the pelvis
- dyspareunia
- pain during defecation or when standing

Diagnosis is a specialist task; patients with CPP ideally require gynecological assessment.

Pharmacotherapy

Pain may respond to simple analgesics such as acetaminophen or naproxen

The management of chronic pelvic pain with opioids could be an option when detailed gynecological assessment has not revealed a pathology that is amenable to treatment

Antidepressants may be helpful, and are frequently prescribed

Physical therapy

Techniques that have been found effective include hot or cold applications, massage, stretching exercises, ultrasound therapy, and transcutaneous electrical nerve stimulation

Psychophysiological therapy

This includes reassurance, counseling, relaxation therapy, stress management programs, and biofeedback techniques. With these, both the frequency and severity of chronic pain can be reduced

Table 6. Management of chronic pelvic pain [21].

"Treatment of pelvic pain is complex in patients with multiple problems. It usually requires specific treatment and simultaneous psychological and physical therapy. Treatment of CPP must be tailored for the individual patient" [21].

Management

Table 6 summarizes treatments that have proved helpful in CPP.

Box 2. Choice of opioid: is oxycodone more effective than morphine in visceral pain?

Recent research suggests that oxycodone, an established synthetic opioid compound, may be more effective than morphine in treating visceral pain. A double-blind randomized study among healthy volunteers (n=24), which compared morphine and oxycodone, found that both opioids were equally effective against a range of experimental pain stimuli in all tissues. However, oxycodone was significantly more effective in the esophagus during mechanical and thermal stimulation ($P<0.001$) [25]. It should be noted that this was a small study group and that the data supporting the greater analgesic efficacy of oxycodone over morphine are as yet experimental.

It has been suggested that oxycodone is effective due to its action at the κ-opioid receptor, while morphine and other μ-agonists often fail to relieve visceral pain. Nalbuphine, pentazocine, and butorphanol are also κ-opioid receptor agonists, but have not been associated with improved analgesic efficacy in visceral pain states.

References

1. Moshiree B, Zhou1 Q, Price DD, et al. Central sensitisation in visceral pain disorders. *Gut* 2006;55:905–8.
2. Patrizi F, Freedman SD, Pascual-Leone A, et al. Novel therapeutic approaches to the treatment of chronic abdominal visceral pain. *Scientific World Journal* 2006;6:472–90.
3. Farthing MJ. Irritable bowel, irritable body, or irritable brain? *BMJ* 1995;310:171–5.
4. American Gastroenterological Association (AGA). AGA technical review on irritable bowel syndrome. *Gastroenterology* 2002;123:2108–31.
5. Hungin AP, Chang L, Locke GR, et al. Irritable bowel syndrome in the United States: prevalence, symptom patterns and impact. *Aliment Pharmacol Ther* 2005;21:1365–75.
6. Whitehead WE, Crowell MD, Robinson JC, et al. Effects of stressful life events on bowel symptoms: subjects with irritable bowel syndrome compared with subjects without bowel dysfunction. *Gut* 1992;33:825–30.
7. Horwitz BL, Lembo AJ, Whitehead WE. Managing irritable bowel syndrome. *Patient Care* 2003;2:18–34.
8. Manning AP, Thompson WG, Heaton KW, et al. Towards positive diagnosis of the irritable bowel. *BMJ* 1978;2:653–4.
9. American Gastroenterological Association medical position statement: irritable bowel syndrome. *Gastroenterology* 2002;123:2105–7.
10. Pain Resource Center. *Menstrual Discomfort.* Available from: www.painresourcecenter.com. Accessed July 30, 2007.
11. French L. Dysmenorrhea. *Am Fam Physician* 2005;71:285–91.
12. Burnett MA, Antao V, Black A, et al. Prevalence of primary dysmenorrhea in Canada. *J Obstet Gynaecol Can* 2005;27:765–70.
13. Coco AS. Primary dysmenorrhea. *Am Fam Physician* 1999;60:689–96.
14. Jamieson DJ, Steege JF. The prevalence of dysmenorrhea, dyspareunia, pelvic pain, and irritable bowel syndrome in primary care practices. *Obstet Gynecol* 1996;87:55–8.
15. Dawood MY. Dysmenorrhea. *Clin Obstet Gynecol* 1990;33:168–78.

16. Proctor M, Murphy P, Pattison H, et al. Behavioural interventions for primary and secondary dysmenorrhoea. *Cochrane Database Syst Rev* 2007;(3):CD002248.

17. Dawood MY. Ibuprofen and dysmenorrhea. *Am J Med* 1984;77:87–94.

18. Marjoribanks J, Proctor ML, Farquhar C. Nonsteroidal anti-inflammatory drugs for primary dysmenorrhoea. *Cochrane Database Syst Rev* 2003;(4):CD001751.

19. Chan FKL. *Primer: Managing NSAID-Induced Ulcer Complications – Balancing Gastrointestinal and Cardiovascular Risks*. Available from www.medscape.com/viewarticle/545617_1. Accessed July 30, 2007.

20. Fortun PJ, Hawkey CJ. Nonsteroidal anti-inflammatory drugs and the small intestine. *Curr Opin Gastroenterol* 2005;21:169–75.

21. Singh MK, Puscheck E. Chronic pelvic pain. *eMedicine*, 2005. Available from: www.emedicine.com/MED/topic2939.htm. Accessed July 30, 2007.

22. Mathias SD, Kuppermann M, Liberman RF. Chronic pelvic pain: prevalence, health-related quality of life, and economic correlates. *Obstet Gynecol* 1996;87:321–7.

23. Haggerty CL, Peipert JF, Weitzen S, et al. Predictors of chronic pelvic pain in an urban population of women with symptoms and signs of pelvic inflammatory disease. *Sex Transm Dis* 2005;32:293–9.

24. Mayo Foundation for Medical Education and Research. *Women's Health. Chronic Pelvic Pain*. Available from: www.mayoclinic.com. Accessed July 30, 2007.

25. Staahl C, Christrup LL, Andersen SD, et al. A comparative study of oxycodone and morphine in a multi-modal, tissue-differentiated experimental pain model. *Pain* 2006;123:28–36.

8 • Neuropathic pain syndromes

Neuropathic pain

Neuropathic pain is defined by the International Association for the Study of Pain (IASP) as: "Pain initiated or caused by a primary lesion or dysfunction of the nervous system [peripheral and/or central]" [1].

Peripheral neuropathic pain

Peripheral neuropathic pain originating from lesions or dysfunction of the peripheral pain pathways can be secondary to multiple causes (eg, diabetes mellitus, cancer, infection, alcohol addiction, autoimmune disease, hereditary factors, congenital factors, neurotoxicity, trauma/structural lesions, paraneoplasia, vitamin deficiencies, or those that are cryptogenic) and multiple biomolecular pathologic mechanisms [2].

Most neuropathic pain conditions develop after partial injuries to peripheral nerves. For example, as observed in animal models of partial nerve injury, both injured and uninjured nociceptor neurons acquire the ability to express genes *de novo* and, therefore, change their phenotype (phenotypic shift). Nociceptor nerve endings develop hypersensitivity to a number of endogenous and environmental factors, such as chemical, mechanical, and thermal stimuli. One example is the upregulation or induction of catecholamine receptors in undamaged nociceptors; in this condition, nociceptors are activated by norepinephrine, and the resulting neuropathic pain has been called sympathetically maintained pain (SMP). Reversal of the phenotypic shift is associated with a reduction in neuropathic pain.

Central neuropathic pain
Central neuropathic pain that originates from lesions or dysfunction of the central nervous system (CNS) pain pathways can also be secondary to multiple causes (eg, spinal cord injury, brain infarction, spinal infarction, syringomyelia, multiple sclerosis) [2] and related to multiple mechanisms (eg, central sensitization, microglial activation, loss of inhibitory interneuron function, abnormal CNS reorganization).

Characteristics of neuropathic pain
Neuropathic pain has certain distinct features [3]:

- It is an ongoing pain that is often described as shooting, stabbing, lancinating, burning, or searing, and is often distinct from nociceptive pain.
- In peripheral neuropathic pain states, pain distribution usually follows an anatomic pattern (eg, stocking-and-glove distribution in peripheral neuropathy, dermatomal distribution in radiculopathy).
- Other signs of sensory or motor dysfunction may be present.

Patients with neuropathic pain may present with some or all of the following abnormal sensory symptoms and signs [2,4]:

- *Paresthesias* – spontaneous, intermittent, painless, abnormal sensations.
- *Dysesthesias* – spontaneous or evoked unpleasant sensations, such as annoying sensations elicited by cold stimuli or pinprick testing.
- *Allodynia* – pain elicited by nonnoxious stimuli (eg, clothing, air movement, tactile stimuli) when applied to the symptomatic cutaneous area. Allodynia can be mechanical (static [eg, induced by the application of a light pressure] or dynamic [eg, induced by moving a soft brush]) or thermal (eg, induced by a nonpainful cold stimulus).

- *Hyperalgesia* – an exaggerated pain response to a mildly noxious (mechanical or thermal) stimulus applied to the symptomatic area.
- *Hyperpathia* – a delayed and explosive pain response to a stimulus applied to the symptomatic area.

Allodynia, hyperalgesia, and hyperpathia represent positive abnormal findings, as opposed to the negative findings of the neurologic sensory examination (ie, hypesthesia and anesthesia) [4]. Heat hyperalgesia and deep mechanical allodynia commonly occur at the cutaneous epicenter of an inflammatory pain generator, also known as the *zone of primary hyperalgesia*. These findings are indicative of peripheral nervous system sensitization, and are related to a local inflammatory state. On the other hand, involvement of the skin surrounding the site of inflammation, also known as the *zone of secondary hyperalgesia*, is indicative of CNS sensitization.

Assessment of neuropathic pain

The successful treatment of neuropathic pain depends on its early identification and classification. The Neuropathic Pain Scale was designed to assess distinct pain qualities associated with neuropathic pain [5]. The scale includes items that assess the global dimensions of pain intensity and pain unpleasantness, and specific qualities of neuropathic pain. This scale can also be used for follow-up assessments.

Investigations

A number of painful neuropathies can present with a variety of complaints. Urinary frequency, weight loss, fatigue, edema, somnolence, skin discoloration (eg, icterus), fever, persistent cough, dry eyes, joint swelling, skin rash, tremors, gait unsteadiness, nail changes, and hair loss should suggest an underlying systemic medical condition. This condition could be diabetes mellitus, hypothyroidism, chronic renal failure, malabsorption, malignancy, connective tissue diseases, chronic infections, use of illicit drugs, alcoholism, abnormal dietary habits, or chronic intoxication (see **Table 1**).

Cause	Example
Metabolic and endocrine disorders	Diabetic neuropathies Hepatic disease Renal disease and hemodialysis Hypothyroidism
Infections	Human immunodeficiency virus Varicella zoster virus Hepatitis B and C virus Human T-cell lymphotropic virus Leprosy Lyme disease
Demyelinating inflammatory disorders	Guillain–Barré syndrome
Malignancies	Multiple myeloma
Entrapment neuropathies	Carpal tunnel syndrome
Connective tissue diseases, granuloma-related disorders, and vasculitides	Sjögren's syndrome Systemic lupus erythematosus (see **Figure 1**) Rheumatoid arthritis Sarcoidosis Polyarteritis nodosa Churg–Strauss vasculitis Wegener's granulomatosis Giant-cell arteritis or temporal arteritis
Immunoglobulinemias	Monoclonal proteins Primary and secondary amyloidosis Cryoglobulinemia
Dietary or absorption abnormalities	Alcoholic neuropathy Celiac disease B_{12}, thiamine, and other vitamin deficiencies Strachan's syndrome
Toxic neuropathies	Heavy metals Chemotherapeutic agents
Hereditary neuropathies	Charcot-Marie-Tooth disease Fabry's disease Familial amyloid polyneuropathy Porphyric neuropathy
Cryptogenic painful neuropathies	Idiopathic polyneuropathy Complex regional pain syndromes Essential trigeminal and glossopharyngeal neuralgias Cryptogenic brachial plexus neuropathy

Table 1. Etiologies of painful peripheral neuropathies [2,4,6,7].

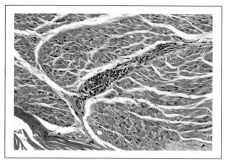

Figure 1. Lymphocytes infiltrating a nerve axon in a patient with polyneuropathy due to systemic lupus erythematosus. A nerve biopsy showed discrete sleeves of lymphocytes around epineurial and perineurial vessels.

Reproduced with permission from Bilbao JM, University of Toronto (*Subacute Multi-System Disorder and Polyneuropathy*. Available from: path.upmc.edu/cases/case202.html).

It is important to screen patients with a chronic neuropathy of undetermined etiology, particularly individuals aged >60 years, for monoclonal proteins; a proportion of these patients may be affected by monoclonal gammopathies. Several autoantibodies with reactivity to various components of the peripheral nerve have been associated with peripheral neuropathies. However, despite all diagnostic efforts, chronic neuropathies of idiopathic origin affect up to 30% of these patients.

Nerve and skin biopsies

The sural nerve is usually selected for biopsy because the sensory deficit following the procedure is limited to a small area along the dorsolateral aspect of the ankle and foot. The biopsy is useful for the diagnosis of vasculitis, amyloidosis, sarcoidosis, immunoglobulin M monoclonal gammopathies, Charcot-Marie-Tooth disease, chronic inflammatory demyelinating polyneuropathies, and small-fiber neuropathies.

Skin biopsy can be used to evaluate the density of unmyelinated fibers within the dermis and epidermis. Immunostaining with the panaxonal marker protein gene product 9.5 has been used to demonstrate the intraepidermal network of C fibers. Patients with diabetic sensory neuropathies, idiopathic neuropathies, and human immune deficiency virus-associated neuropathies have been found to have a significantly diminished intraepidermal density of small fibers.

Electrodiagnostic studies

Electromyography (EMG) and nerve conduction velocity (NCV) studies help to localize the lesion and can indicate an axonal versus a focal segmental demyelinating process. For example, the EMG–NCV study might identify a radiculopathy or mononeuropathy, ie, a focal process affecting a specific root or nerve. Common causes of mononeuropathy include a traumatic injury, compression or nerve entrapment, ischemia, and cancer.

The study might also reveal a *mononeuropathy multiplex*, a pathology of multiple but noncontiguous nerves. Mononeuropathy multiplex is often the result of vasculitis and microangiopathy causing axonal disease in multiple non-contiguous nerves. EMG–NCV studies can also help to detect diffuse abnormalities, indicating a polyneuropathy. Of note, diabetes mellitus, hypothyroidism, and hereditary neuropathy with liability to pressure palsy can all cause neuropathies that predispose affected patients to develop superimposed entrapment neuropathies.

Diabetic neuropathy

Diabetic neuropathy can be defined as a group of peripheral somatic and autonomic nerve disorders that are associated with diabetes mellitus. Diabetic neuropathy is the leading cause of foot ulcers, which, in turn, are a major cause of amputation. Painful diabetic neuropathy affects symmetric body areas; generally the feet, but sometimes also the hands.

Epidemiology

It has been estimated that 20–24% of diabetic Americans experience painful diabetic neuropathy [8]. In addition, 21.5% of those with undiagnosed diabetes have been found to

Symptoms	Description
Sensory	Symptoms include painful sensations (burning, pricking, electrical sensations, squeezing, constricting) or nonpainful sensations (numbness, tingling, feeling of wearing gloves, walking on stilts)
Motor	Distal symptoms include impaired fine coordination (eg, difficulty in opening tins, toe dragging on walking) Proximal weakness may include difficulty with climbing stairs, or with rising from a lying or sitting position
Autonomic	These can be: • sudomotor: dry skin, lack of sweating • pupillary: sensitivity to bright lights • cardiovascular: postural hypotension • GI: nocturnal diarrhea, constipation • urologic: urinary retention • sexual: impotence, ejaculatory dysfunction

Table 2. Symptoms of diabetic neuropathy [10]. GI: gastrointestinal.

have a positive screening test for peripheral neuropathy [9]. Risk factors probably include a longer duration of diabetes mellitus and poor glycemic control [8].

Clinical presentation

- In type 1 diabetes, distal polyneuropathy usually becomes apparent after many years of prolonged hyperglycemia.
- In type 2 diabetes, neuropathy tends to present after only a few years of poorly controlled hyperglycemia.
- Early diabetic polyneuropathy is frequently missed. The physician should therefore examine the patient proactively and systematically for symptoms.

Symptoms can be divided into somatic (sensory, motor) and autonomic (see **Table 2**) [10].

Diagnosis

Painful diabetic neuropathy is diagnosed mainly based on the history and physical examination. The main differential pain diagnoses are listed in **Table 3**.

Condition	Key characteristics
Claudication	Usually intermittent, remitting with rest; other features suggest arterial insufficiency
Osteoarthritis	Pain is usually gradual in onset and in one or two joints
	Morning stiffness; pain worsens with exercise and improves with rest
Radiculopathy	Can result from disc herniation or spondylotic disease of the spine
	Magnetic resonance imaging of the lumbosacral spine can localize the lesion site
Plantar fasciitis	Pain in the plantar region of the foot; pain with each step; worsens with prolonged activity
Tarsal tunnel syndrome	Caused by entrapment of the posterior tibial nerve
	Pain and numbness from beneath the medial malleolus to the sole
	Nerve conduction studies and magnetic resonance imaging may be helpful in diagnosis
Vitamin B_{12} deficiency	Comorbid hematologic (eg, megaloblastic anemia, pancytopenia) or psychiatric (eg, confusion, dementia) signs may be present
	Diagnosed on hematology
Erythromelalgia	Burning pain and bright red color of toes, feet, and hands in association with ambient temperature changes
	Relieved by cold temperature, immersion of the limbs in cold water, or application of ice packs
	The pain is made worse by hot ambient temperature

Table 3. Differential pain diagnosis: common pain syndromes with presentations similar to that of diabetic peripheral neuropathic pain [11].

"When assessing patients with diabetes mellitus, a simple yet key question to ask is: 'Do your feet burn, hurt, or tingle?' A positive answer is highly suggestive of diabetic peripheral neuropathic pain (DPNP). Although DPNP is the most likely diagnosis in these patients, other potential causes of DPNP exist that must be excluded before the DPNP diagnosis can be made" [11].

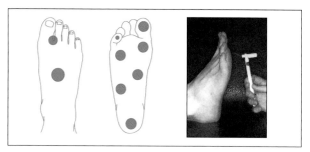

Figure 2. The monofilament test for diabetic neuropathy.

The following confirmatory neurologic tests may be applied [12]:

- a comprehensive foot examination, which involves the assessment of protective sensation with a nylon monofilament (see **Figure 2**)
- vibratory thresholds using a tuning fork
- NCV studies
- EMG, testing the response of the muscles to nerve signals
- quantitative sensory testing, which uses the response to stimuli (eg, pressure, vibration, temperature) to assess sensory thresholds
- ultrasound (eg, to check bladder function)
- heart rate variability testing (R-R interval) to assess the electrocardiographic response to deep breathing, Valsalva maneuver, and changes in posture (early signs)

Management and general measures
- The patient must maintain tight glycemic control. Monitoring of hemoglobin A_{1c} is valuable in assessing the long-term stability of glycemic control.
- Any patient with evidence of diabetic neuropathy should be considered at risk of foot ulceration. It is important to educate each patient on foot care or to refer him/her to a podiatrist. Preventive and symptomatic treatments include foot care, weight reduction, and sensible footwear.
- Regular examination, including skin and foot inspection, is vital.

Class	Examples	Typical doses[a]
Tricyclic drugs	Amitriptyline	10–75 mg at bedtime
	Nortriptyline	25–75 mg at bedtime
	Imipramine	25–75 mg at bedtime
Anticonvulsants	Gabapentin	300–1,200 mg TID
	Carbamazepine	200–400 mg TID
	Pregabalin	100 mg TID
5-hydroxytryptamine and norepinephrine uptake inhibitor	Duloxetine	60–120 mg daily
TRPV1 receptors	Capsaicin cream	0.025–0.075% applied TID–QID

Table 4. Drugs that may be used in the treatment of painful diabetic neuropathy. [a]Dose response may vary; initial doses need to be low and titrated up. TID: three times daily; QID: four times daily.

Reproduced with permission from the American Diabetes Association (Position statement. Standards of medical care in diabetes – 2007. *Diab Care* 2007;30:S4–41).

- Patients with leg weakness might require sticks, crutches, or a walking frame; these are best prescribed by a physical therapist.
- Simple splints, constraining movement, can help weak wrist extension.
- Disabled patients will require help from a multidisciplinary team, including an occupational therapist who can advise on special utensils and home adaptations.

A 2007 position statement by the American Diabetes Association recommends the medications shown in **Table 4** for the treatment of symptomatic diabetic neuropathy [13].

Combination therapy

There is some evidence for the efficacy of combined medications in painful diabetic neuropathy.

- Gilron et al. (2005) found that, in 35 patients with diabetic neuropathy and 22 with postherpetic neuralgia (PHN), a combination of gabapentin and morphine achieved better analgesia at lower doses than did each as a single drug. Constipation, sedation, and dry mouth were the most frequent adverse effects [14].

- An analysis of clinical trial data has indicated that the intensity of neuropathic pain gradually increases throughout the day. This pattern was preserved during treatment with gabapentin, morphine, or a combination of the two. The researchers concluded that recognition of such patterns may guide treatment strategies such as the targeted timing of analgesic therapies [15].

Case study[a]

A 63-year-old man with diabetes has had burning pain in both feet for several months. It is much worse at night, but also limits walking during the day. His only other health problem is benign prostatic hyperplasia. On examination, he has absent Achilles tendon reflexes, absent sensitivity to light rubbing of the feet, and symmetric loss of pinprick and vibratory sensation from his toes to mid-shin.

It is clear that this patient has developed neuropathic pain. The presence of diabetes suggests the diagnosis, and the burning quality and nocturnal worsening of the pain indicate a neuropathic process.

Treatment should begin with optimization of glucose control. Next, local measures should be used where possible. Capsaicin cream might be successful, but the patient may be unable to tolerate the cream's initial burning because of allodynia. Comfortable footwear should be recommended, with an insole of silicon or similar material. Such seemingly simple rehabilitative measures can often make a big difference.

The mainstay of treatment should be pharmacologic methods. Treatment should be started with a gabapentinoid (gabapentin, pregabalin), titrated to provide adequate pain relief. The use of an antidepressant and/or opioid analgesic as single-agent or combination therapy may be considered.

[a]Abridged with permission from McGraw-Hill (Belgrade MJ. Following the clues to neuropathic pain. Distribution and other leads reveal the cause and the treatment approach. *Postgrad Med* 1999;106:127–40).

Age ≥50 years

Greater severity of acute pain during zoster

More severe rash

Prodromal pain before onset of the rash

Patients with all of these risk factors have a 50–75% risk of persisting pain

Table 5. Risk factors for postherpetic neuralgia [10].

Postherpetic neuralgia

Herpes zoster (shingles) results from the reactivation of latent varicella zoster virus (VZV) from the dorsal root ganglion or cranial nerve ganglia, present since a primary infection with varicella (chicken pox), usually in childhood. The VZV manifestation can cause extensive inflammatory, hemorrhagic, and necrotic changes in the dorsal root ganglia, as well as in the corresponding dorsal horns of the spinal cord.

PHN (pain that persists at least 3 months after the acute rash of herpes zoster heals) is the most common and feared complication of the disorder. PHN may cause fatigue, insomnia, depression, anxiety, interference with social roles and leisure activity, and impaired basic and instrumental activities of daily living [8].

Epidemiology
- Herpes zoster affects an estimated 800,000 people each year, most of whom are elderly or immunosuppressed [8].
- Between 25% and 50% of herpes zoster patients aged >50 years develop PHN, depending on early antiviral therapy for herpes zoster [8].
- The risk of developing herpes zoster has been observed to increase sharply with age, and PHN tends to be more frequent and severe in older individuals [16].
- The risk of PHN is highly variable (see **Table 5**).

Management
In order to reduce the risk of PHN, all patients with ongoing herpes zoster should be treated as early as possible for the

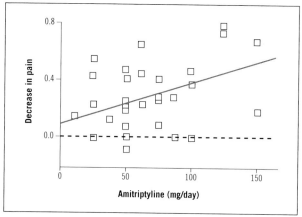

Figure 3. Reduction of pain with amitriptyline in 58 patients with postherpetic neuralgia over 6 weeks.

Reproduced with permission from Lippincott Williams & Wilkins (Max MB, Schafer SC, Culnane M, et al. Amitriptyline, but not lorazepam, relieves postherpetic neuralgia. *Neurology* 1988;38:1427–32).

acute symptoms, especially patients aged ≥50 years, who are at much higher risk.

Antiviral drugs

Antiviral drugs such as acyclovir, famciclovir, and valacyclovir hasten rash healing, reduce acute pain, and reduce the risk of PHN by approximately 50% [17]. However, 20% of patients aged >50 years who are treated with famciclovir or valaciclovir still report pain at 6 months [18,19].

Pain management

Classes of pharmacologic agents with established efficacy for PHN pain are [20]:

- tricyclic antidepressants (eg, amitriptyline) (see **Figure 3**)
- gabapentinoids (eg, gabapentin, pregabalin)
- opioids (eg, morphine, oxycodone, methadone)
- topical analgesics and anesthetics (eg, lidocaine 5% patch)

Aspirin in cream and capsaicin are also possibly effective, but are likely to have a low magnitude of benefit [20].

Complex regional pain syndrome

In 1864, the American Silas Weir Mitchell, who was considered the most eminent neurologist of his time, described a painful condition that he termed 'causalgia'. He observed the syndrome, which consisted of burning pain and trophic changes, in wounded veterans of the American Civil War. This clinical pain state, which has since been called by many names, continues to perplex medical scientists and practitioners.

In 1900, the German orthopedist Paul Sudeck described a painful condition occurring after a minor injury (eg, a sprain). This condition was associated with bone atrophy, particularly of the carpal and tarsal bones.

In 1916, the French Surgeon René Leriche argued that causalgia was due to "pain from irritation of the sympathetic nerves" and was alleviated by sympathectomy. In 1946, J Evans observed that pain could be relieved by a sympathetic blockade, and introduced the popular term 'reflex sympathetic dystrophy' (RSD).

RSD became the predominant nomenclature, although subsequent investigations and observations proved that only a subgroup of cases diagnosed as RSD were maintained by the activity of the sympathetic nervous system. In addition, it was noted that some patients with a history of RSD did not have dystrophic features.

In 1994, the International Association for the Study of Pain renamed 'RSD' as 'complex regional pain syndrome (CRPS) type 1' and 'causalgia' as 'CRPS type 2' (see **Table 6**).

Following a distal limb traumatic injury and subsequent limb immobilization (often an important predisposing factor in the medical history of this disorder), some patients develop CRPS. Trigger mechanisms for CRPS include:

- trauma
- limb immobilization
- ischemia/reperfusion
- genetic factors

CRPS type 1 (reflex sympathetic dystrophy)

1. The presence of an initiating noxious event or a cause of immobilization

2. Continuing pain, allodynia, or hyperalgesia with which the pain is disproportionate to the inciting event

3. Evidence at some time of edema, changes in skin blood flow, or abnormal sudomotor (sweat gland) activity in the painful region

4. The diagnosis is excluded by the existence of conditions that would otherwise account for the degree of pain and dysfunction

Criteria 2,3, and 4 are necessary for a diagnosis of CRPS (1 is not always present)

CRPS type 2 (causalgia)

1. The presence of continuing pain, allodynia, or hyperalgesia after a nerve injury, not necessarily limited to the distribution of the injured nerve

2. Evidence at some time of edema, changes in skin blood flow, or abnormal sudomotor activity in the region of the pain

3. The diagnosis is excluded by the existence of conditions that would otherwise account for the degree of pain and dysfunction

All three criteria must be satisfied

Table 6. Complex regional pain syndrome (CRPS) diagnosis: the four International Association for the Study of Pain criteria.

Adapted with permission from the IASP (Merskey H, Bodguk N, Editors. *Classification of Chronic Pain: Descriptions of Chronic Pain Syndromes and Definitions of Pain Terms*, 2nd edn. Seattle: IASP Press, 1994:40–3).

CRPS can be secondary to an abnormal neuroimmunologic inflammatory process. An outgrowth of this concept is the number of observations addressing the role of macrophages and macrophage-released cytokines, as well as tissue-released nerve growth factor (NGF) (eg, from mast cells, fibroblasts, keratinocytes) in the genesis of hyperalgesia. Specific inflammatory cytokines (eg, tumor necrosis factor-α, interleukin-1β), in combination with tissue-released growth factors (eg, NGF), are known to not only bring on hyperalgesia by sensitizing tissue nociceptors, but also, possibly, to initiate altered gene expression in primary sensory pain neurons (eg, changes in sodium channels and expression of altered receptors and channels, including adrenoreceptor excitability). The end result is a chronic neuropathic pain condition.

Neurotrophic factors, including NGF, can induce miniature axon sprouts from both the endings of afferent fibers and the sympathetic efferent nerves, perhaps favoring a coupling between somatic and sympathetic nerves. In this context, norepinephrine, released locally from the sympathetic efferents, would activate the altered nociceptors expressing adrenoreceptor excitability.

α-Adrenoreceptor excitability represents the pathophysiologic basis of SMP. SMP can complicate the pathogenesis of CRPS, but might well be a reversible phenomenon in the course of CRPS. In several instances, CRPS has appeared to be maintained by plastic mechanisms (eg, the SMP mechanism) that can be switched off by early and aggressive therapeutic interventions. It is conceivable that SMP can complicate not only CRPS but also other painful disorders, including shingles, neuralgias, and metabolic or autoimmune neuropathies.

Management
The contemporary treatment of CRPS calls for an aggressive, sophisticated, multimodal approach. This should include a combination of pharmacologic interventions and physical therapy, and, when clinically indicated, psychological interventions.

Current expert opinion, which is based on preliminary data from recent animal and human studies, as well as on collective clinical experience, recommends that both aggressive multidisciplinary approaches and individualized treatment strategies be used in the management of CRPS. Thus, as soon as the diagnosis of CRPS is entertained, early specialized consultation should be obtained. Early and aggressive pharmacologic and procedural interventions should be instituted for pain control; and physical and rehabilitation treatments should be instituted to avert limb immobilization, tissue concentration of free radicals, contractures, and muscle atrophies.

At present, there is no Food and Drug Administration-approved medication for this condition. The field of CRPS pharmacotherapy presents a paucity of randomized controlled

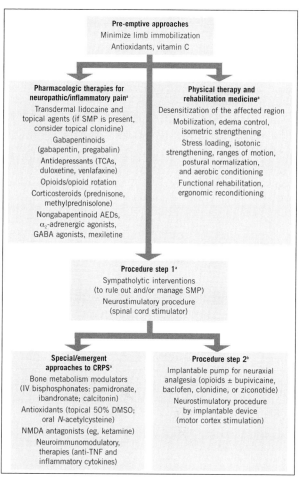

Figure 4. Treatment algorithm for complex regional pain syndrome (CRPS). AED: antiepileptic drug; DMSO: dimethyl sulfoxide; GABA: γ-aminobutyric acid; SMP: sympathetically maintained pain; TCA: tricyclic antidepressant; TNF: tumor necrosis factor.

[a]While balancing safety, benefit, and patient tolerability to medications, various pharmacologic treatments, physical therapy, and interventional approaches can be combined to achieve the most satisfactory outcome of improvement in pain and function. On a compassionate basis and according to the physician's experience, the patient's clinical condition, and the patient's previous response to more conventional treatments, off-label emergent approaches to refractory CRPS may be possible; these include empirical trials of one or more of the topical, oral, or parenteral emergent therapies. [b]Intrathecal baclofen is recommended for refractory CRPS-associated dystonia. On a compassionate basis, motor cortex stimulation can be considered.

Adapted with permission from Begell House (Pappagallo M, Knotkova H, DeNardis L. The multifaceted CRPS/RSD: emerging mechanisms and therapy. *Critical Reviews in Physical and Rehabilitation Medicine* 2006;18:257–82).

trials, a large variety of anecdotal observations, and off-label treatments of unclear benefit; however, novel treatments are under investigation.

The management of CRPS is usually a challenge. The use of conventional agents for neuropathic and inflammatory pain, in combination with emergent pharmacologic interventions on a compassionate basis, represents a new trend in the contemporary approach for poorly responsive CRPS (see **Figure 4**) [21].

References

1. International Association for the Study of Pain (IASP). *IASP Pain Terminology*. Available from www.iasp-pain.org. Accessed July 30, 2007.

2. Baron R. Mechanisms of disease: neuropathic pain – a clinical perspective. *Nat Clin Pract Neurol* 2006;2:95–106.

3. Institute for Clinical Systems Improvement (ICSI). *Assessment and Management of Chronic Pain*. Bloomington: ICSI, 2007. Available from: www.icsi.org. Accessed August 30, 2007.

4. Dworkin RH, Backonja M, Rowbotham MC, et al. Advances in neuropathic pain: diagnosis, mechanisms, and treatment recommendations. *Arch Neurol* 2003;60:1524–34.

5. Galer BS, Jensen MP. Development and preliminary validation of a pain measure specific to neuropathic pain: the Neuropathic Pain Scale. *Neurology* 1997;48:332–8.

6. Hughes RA. Regular review. Peripheral neuropathy. *BMJ* 2002;324:466–9.

7. Dworkin RH, Backonja M, Rowbotham MC, et al. Advances in neuropathic pain: diagnosis, mechanisms, and treatment recommendations. *Arch Neurol* 2003;60:1524–34.

8. Schmader KE. Epidemiology and impact on quality of life of postherpetic neuralgia and painful diabetic neuropathy. *Clin J Pain* 2002;18:350–4.

9. Koopman RJ, Mainous AG 3rd, Liszka HA, et al. Evidence of nephropathy and peripheral neuropathy in US adults with undiagnosed diabetes. *Ann Fam Med* 2006;4:427–32.

10. Dworkin RH, Schmader KE. Epidemiology and natural history of herpes zoster and postherpetic neuralgia. In: Watson CPN, Gershon AA, Editors. *Herpes Zoster and Postherpetic Neuralgia*, 2nd edn. New York: Elsevier, 2001:39–64.

11. Argoff CE, Cole BE, Fishbain DA, et al. Diabetic peripheral neuropathic pain: clinical and quality-of-life issues. *Mayo Clin Proc* 2006;81(4 Suppl.):S3–11.

12. Aring AM, Jones DE, Falko JM. Evaluation and prevention of diabetic neuropathy. *Am Fam Physician* 2005;71:2123–8.

13. Boulton AJ, Vinik AI, Arezzo JC, et al. Diabetic neuropathies. A statement by the American Diabetes Association. *Diab Care* 2005;28:956–62.

14. Gilron I, Bailey JM, Tu D, et al. Morphine, gabapentin, or their combination for neuropathic pain. *N Engl J Med* 2005;352:1324–34.

15. Odrich M, Bailey JM, Cahill CM, et al. Chronobiological characteristics of painful diabetic neuropathy and postherpetic neuralgia: diurnal pain variation and effects of analgesic therapy. *Pain* 2006;120:207–12.

16. Insinga RP, Itzler RF, Pellissier JM, et al. The incidence of herpes zoster in a United States administrative database. *J Gen Intern Med* 2005;20:748–53.

17. Cunningham AL, Dworkin RH. The management of post-herpetic neuralgia. *BMJ* 2000;321:778–9.

18. Beutner KR, Friedman DJ, Forszpaniak C, et al. Valaciclovir compared with acyclovir for improved therapy for herpes zoster in immunocompetent adults. *Antimicrob Agents Chemother* 1995;39:1546–53.

19. Dworkin RH, Boon RJ, Griffin DR, et al. Postherpetic neuralgia: impact of famciclovir, age, rash severity and acute pain in herpes zoster patients. *J Infect Dis* 1998;178(Suppl.1):S76–80.

20. Dubinsky RM, Kabbani H, El-Chami Z, et al. Practice parameter: treatment of postherpetic neuralgia. An evidence-based report of the Quality Standards Subcommittee of the American Academy of Neurology. *Neurology* 2004;63:959–65.

21. Pappagallo M, Knotkova H, DeNardis L. The multifaceted CRPS/RSD: emerging mechanisms and therapy. *Critical Reviews in Physical and Rehabilitation Medicine* 2006;18:257–82.

9 • Headache

In 1988, the International Headache Society (IHS) provided a detailed classification of headache (with minor revisions in 2004) upon which most clinicians and researchers have subsequently relied [1,2]. The IHS defined 14 general groupings of headache disorders, with numerous subgroups. Many of these, however – mainly types of secondary headache – are rarely encountered in routine practice.

For most clinical purposes, headache can be broadly grouped as shown in **Table 1** [2].

> "Primary headache is treated symptomatically, with the goal being relief and preventing recurrence. Although secondary headache may also require symptomatic relief, treatment of the underlying disease process is the focus of care" [3].

Headache assessment

The vital first step in the assessment of headache is to determine whether the headache is primary (ie, tension, migraine, or cluster) or secondary to an underlying cause. Red flags (see **Table 2**) are normally an indication for referral and/or neuroimaging (computed tomography or magnetic resonance image scanning) [4].

Type of headache	Description
Primary	No apparent underlying disease process: • tension-type headache • cluster headache • migraine
Secondary	Attributed to an underlying organic disease and a symptom of a recognized disease process, eg, headache due to: • head or neck trauma • cranial or cervical vascular disorder • nonvascular intracranial disorder • a substance or its withdrawal • infection • disturbance of homeostasis • a disorder of facial or cranial structures • psychiatric disorder

Table 1. Types of headache [2].

Indicators of possible serious underlying pathology include:
• a new or different headache
• 'thunderclap' headache (peak intensity within seconds to minutes)
• worst headache ever
• focal neurologic signs or symptoms (eg, papilledema, motor weakness, memory loss, papillary abnormalities, sensory loss)
• change in existing headaches
• new-onset headache at age >50 years
• headache associated with systemic symptoms (eg, fever, weight loss, jaw claudication)

Table 2. Red flag signs in headache.

Reproduced with permission from the National Headache Foundation (*Standards of Care for Headache Diagnosis and Treatment*, 2004).

Patient history information should include [3,4]:

- the course and duration of symptoms (a headache diary is often helpful)
- the quality of the headache (eg, steady, pounding, stabbing)
- the intensity, perhaps using a visual analog scale

- Avoid drug overuse; analgesics and other drugs used to treat headache can result in medication-overuse headache.

Pharmacologic therapy

Most patients with tension-type headache use analgesics (98% in one study), eg, acetaminophen (56%), aspirin (17%) [11].

Studies (mainly randomized controlled trials) indicate that the following are effective in tension-type headache [3]:

- nonsteroidal anti-inflammatory drugs (NSAIDs), including ibuprofen (may be more effective than acetaminophen) and ketoprofen
- acetaminophen

Analgesics can be augmented with a sedating antihistamine (eg, diphenhydramine) or with an antiemetic (eg, metoclopramide), depending on the individual's symptoms (eg, anxiety, restlessness, frequent nausea).

Amitriptyline and serotonin and norepinephrine reuptake inhibitors (eg, venlafaxine) may be effective in prophylaxis, as may smoking cessation. Prophylactic therapy should be reserved for patients with frequent tension-type headache (>15 headaches per month) [12].

Nonpharmacologic therapy

Reports suggest that the following therapies may be helpful, although large trials of their roles in tension-type headache are lacking [3,13]:

- biofeedback
- relaxation therapy
- self-hypnosis
- cognitive therapy
- acupuncture

Some of these treatments are addressed in more detail in **Chapter 17**.

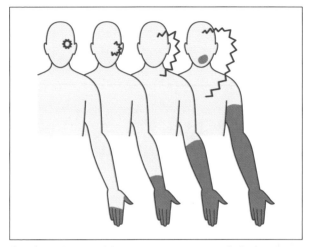

Figure 3. Development of the two most common auras of migraine, scintillating scotoma and digitolingual paresthesia.

Reproduced with permission from Mosby (Carlson K, Editor. *Primary Care of Women*. Mosby, 1995).

Migraine

Migraine is a chronic neurologic disorder characterized by episodic attacks of head pain and associated symptoms [5]. The headache may be unilateral or bilateral, and is frequently associated with nausea and vomiting. Some migraine headaches are accompanied by a prodromal aura, which frequently consists of neurologic symptoms, eg, dizziness, tinnitus, scotomata, photophobia, or visual scintillations (bright zigzag lines) [14].

The disorder is usually subdivided into migraine with and without aura (see **Figure 3**), and probable migraine [5]. Migraine without aura is more common, accounting for approximately 80% of cases [14,15].

Epidemiology

In a survey of 162,576 participants (aged ≥12 years), the American Migraine Prevalence and Prevention Study reported the following results [16]:

Symptom	Description
Headache	Moderate to severe intensity, with or without aura (see below)
	Most are unilateral, but 30–40% are bilateral
	Described as throbbing or pulsatile, lasting 4–72 hours
Aura (in 20%)	Begins and ends prior to the headache
	Visual aura symptoms are the most common, eg:
	• scotomata
	• fortification spectra (bright, shimmering, jagged lines that can spread across the visual field)
	• hallucinations (usually visual, although auditory hallucinations have also been described)
Systemic manifestations	Nausea (80–90%), vomiting (40–60%), photophobia (80%)
Triggers	Common precipitating factors include:
	• menstruation
	• stress
	• lack of sleep
	• strenuous exercise
	• certain foods (eg, cheese, chocolate, red wine)
Keeping a symptom diary can be helpful in subsequent management	

Table 4. History and symptoms of migraine [4,14,17].

- The prevalence of migraine was 17.1% in females and 5.6% in males.
- Only 56.2% of those with migraine had ever received a medical diagnosis.
- Migraine peaked in middle life, and was lower in adolescents and those aged >60 years.
- Of those who experienced migraine, 31.3% had an attack frequency of three or more migraines per month; 53.7% reported severe impairment or the need for bed rest.

Diagnosis

The basic principles of diagnosis are as for all headaches (see 'Headache assessment'), in that the prime requirement is the exclusion of secondary headache, with vigilance for red flags. Otherwise, migraine is diagnosed largely on the history (see **Table 4**). Further investigations are normally required only if a differential diagnosis is suspected.

Management

Most migraine patients can be effectively treated with various acute headache medications (eg, aspirin, NSAIDs, triptans) [12] and nonpharmacologic strategies (eg, lifestyle regulation, stimulant reduction, trigger avoidance). However, the following clinical presentations warrant the introduction of a pharmacologic agent to reduce the frequency, duration, and severity of migraine attacks [18]:

- Headache frequency >2 days/week or >8 days/month.
- Use of acute medications (whether or not successful) >2 days/week.
- Headache attacks that remain disabling despite aggressive acute intervention, as documented by lifestyle interference, ratings on disability scales, or use of rescue medications more than once a month.
- Presence of prolonged aura (>1 hour), complex aura (basilar or hemiplegic), or migraine-induced stroke.
- Contraindications to, failure of, overuse of, or adverse events with acute therapies.
- Patient desire to reduce frequency of acute attacks.

The US Headache Consortium has developed guidelines for the prevention of migraine [19]. Group 1 and 2 medications are shown in **Table 5**. Therapy should be initiated at the lowest effective dose, and increased slowly until clinical benefit is achieved or until limited by adverse events. The effects of therapy should be monitored through the use of a headache diary. The full guideline is available from the American Headache Society, at www.americanheadachesociety.org.

Cluster headache

Cluster headaches are attacks of severe, unilateral pain that last 15–180 minutes and occur from once every other day to eight times a day. The headache can be orbital, supraorbital, and/or temporal [2]:

Group	Medication
Group 1: Medium to high efficacy, good strength of evidence, and a range of severity (mild to moderate) and frequency (infrequent to frequent) of side effects	Amitriptyline (10–150 mg/day)
	Divalproex sodium (250–500 mg/day)
	Timolol (10–20 mg/day)
	Propranolol (20–120 mg/day)
	Topiramate (50–150 mg/day)[a]
Group 2: Lower efficacy than those listed above, or limited strength of evidence, and mild to moderate side effects	Atenolol
	Gabapentin
	Metoprolol
	Nadolol
	Naproxen
	Nimodipine
	Verapamil
	Botulinum toxin

Table 5. US Headache Consortium guidelines for migraine prophylaxis: group 1 and 2 medications [19]. [a]Based on evidence not available at the time of guideline publication.

- The episodic type is characterized by attacks that occur in periods lasting 7 days to 1 year, separated by pain-free intervals lasting ≥1 month [2].
- The chronic form is characterized by the absence of these pain-free intervals. Chronic cluster headache can arise *de novo* or develop from the episodic type [2].

Epidemiology
- Cluster headache affects 0.1% of adults [20].
- It is more common in males, in the ratio of 2:1, although this ratio appears to be equalizing [21].
- Patients often first experience cluster headache in their 20s (see **Figure 4**) [21]. Peak onset may be later in women [22].
- Ethnic differences in prevalence have not been studied.
- Smoking, head injury, shift work, and a family history of headache have all been associated with cluster headache [22].
- A number of factors can trigger episodes of pain, including alcohol, stress, exposure to heat or cold, and certain foods (eg, eggs, dairy products) [22].

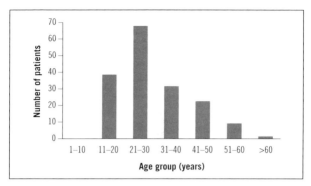

Figure 4. Age at onset of episodic cluster headache among 180 patients.

Reproduced with permission from Blackwell (Manzoni GC, Terzano MG, Bono G, et al. Cluster headache – clinical findings in 180 patients. *Cephalalgia* 1983;3:21–30).

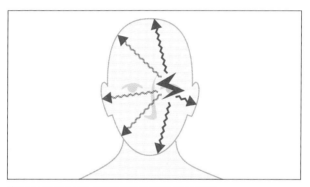

Figure 5. Typical pain distribution in cluster headache.

Clinical features and characteristics of pain

The pain usually begins in, around, or above the eye or the temple (see **Figure 5**). The attacks are accompanied by one or more of the following features, all of which are ipsilateral [2]:

* conjunctival injection and/or lacrimation
* nasal congestion and/or rhinorrhea
* forehead and facial sweating
* eyelid edema
* miosis and/or ptosis
* restlessness or agitation

Acute treatment	The first-line treatments for acute cluster headache are oxygen or sumatriptan, or a combination of the two
	Less well-studied alternatives for acute treatment include intranasal dihydroergotamine, intranasal lidocaine, and intranasal capsaicin
Prophylaxis	Verapamil 240 mg/day can effectively reduce the number of attacks during a cluster headache period
	Less well-studied alternatives for prophylaxis include prednisone and antiepileptic drugs; these should only be considered if verapamil is not tolerated or not effective

Table 6. Key clinical recommendations for cluster headache [23].

Diagnosis

The basic principles of diagnosis are as for all headaches (see 'Headache assessment'), with vigilance for red flags.

Management

There has been little research into behavior and lifestyle interventions in cluster headache, but it has been suggested that treatments that are effective in other type of pain (eg, biofeedback, cognitive therapy; see **Chapter 17**) could be of value [23]. Where medications are concerned, Beck et al. have set out evidence-based recommendations, summarized in **Table 6**.

The most effective treatments for acute attacks include oxygen inhalation (100% for 10–15 minutes at the onset of an attack), subcutaneous sumatriptan, and dihydroergotamine [12]. Maintenance prophylaxis is extremely important; verapamil is first-line. The patient should also be advised to avoid alcohol during the cluster period [12].

Case study: cluster headache precipitated by medication[a]

The patient is a man aged 78 years with no previous history of migraine, tension, or cluster headaches. His family history is positive for headache: his mother had suffered from migraine headaches, as does his son. He smoked until age 60 years; he has a history of coronary artery disease, and had a coronary artery bypass graft at age 61 years.

The patient was in his usual state of health until he developed headaches over a 1-week period. The headaches were left-sided, and he described them as, "A red-hot iron from above my eye through to the back." The intensity was severe, with lacrimation on the affected side. The headache would begin 2 hours after he took his morning medication, lasting on average 3 hours. During the pain, he would pace to and fro. Ice and heat did not help.

His medication was isosorbide mononitrate sustained-release 30 mg in the morning, diltiazem sustained-release 120 mg in the morning, pentoxifylline 400 mg in the morning, simvastatin 40 mg at night, doxazosin mesylate 1 mg at night, and aspirin 325 mg and folic acid 400 mg, one of each in the morning.

The patient had a normal neurologic work-up; magnetic resonance angiography revealed a right internal carotid occlusion, an old finding. His endocrine work-up was normal.

Oxygen therapy relieved the headache for 1 week, but soon became ineffective. Botulinum toxin injections, intranasal lidocaine, and hydrocodone/acetaminophen tablets provided no relief. After 3 months of daily headaches, the isosorbide was discontinued. The headaches immediately disappeared, and began again when the medication was restarted. The dose was decreased to 15 mg each morning, which did not result in any headache. For the past year, the patient has remained headache-free.

Comment: The anti-anginal drug isosorbide mononitrate has been known to precipitate headache, although cluster headaches are unusual. Nitroglycerin is known to precipitate cluster headaches.

Medications are often a trigger for headache. This case suggests that medication should be considered as a trigger for new-onset headache, even when the patient has been taking it for many years. In this case, the patient had been taking isosorbide for 10 years.

ᵃAbridged with permission from Robbins Headache Clinic (Robbins L. *Cluster Headache Precipitated By Isosorbide Mononitrate: A Case Report*, 2003. Available from: www.headachedrugs.com/archives/cluster_headache_isosorbide.html).

References

1. Headache Classification Committee of the International Headache Society. Classification and diagnostic criteria for headache disorders, cranial neuralgias and facial pain. *Cephalalgia* 1988;8(Suppl. 7):1–96.

2. Headache Classification Subcommittee of the International Headache Society. The International Classification of Headache Disorders, 2nd edition. *Cephalalgia* 2004;24(Suppl. 1):9–160.

3. Millea PJ, Brodie JJ. Tension-type headache. *Am Fam Physician* 2002;66:797–804.

4. Bal SK, Hollingworth GR. Headache. *BMJ* 2005;330:346.

5. Martin V, Elkind A. Diagnosis and classification of primary headache disorders. In: *Standards of Care for Headache Diagnosis and Treatment*. Chicago: National Headache Foundation, 2004:73–80.

6. Ferri FF, Editor. *Ferri's Clinical Advisor*. St Louis: Mosby, 2005.

7. Dalhousie University, Nova Scotia. *Chronic Daily Headache – Medication-induced Headache. Epidemiology*. Available from: www.digital-fx.ca/cme/neuro/neur-virtprof3.html. Accessed July 30, 2007.

8. Abu-Arefeh I, Russell G. Prevalence of headache and migraine in schoolchildren. *BMJ* 1994;309:765–9.

9. Ashina M, Bendtsen L, Jensen R, et al. Muscle hardness in patients with chronic tension-type headache: relation to actual headache state. *Pain* 1999;79:201–5.

10. Ashina M, Bendtsen L, Jensen R, et al. Nitric oxide-induced headache in patients with chronic tension-type headache. *Brain* 2000;123:1830–7.

11. Spira PJ. Tension headache. *Aust Fam Physician* 1998;27:597–600.

12. Institute for Clinical Systems Improvement (ICSI). *Diagnosis and Treatment of Headache*. Bloomington: ICSI, 2006. Available from: www.icsi.org. Accessed August 30, 2007.

13. Mauskop A, Graff-Radford S. Special treatment situations: alternative headache treatments. In: *Standards of Care for Headache Diagnosis and Treatment*. Chicago: National Headache Foundation, 2004:115–22.

14. Blanda M, Wright J. Headache, migraine. *eMedicine*. Available from: www.emedicine.com/EMERG/topic230.htm. Accessed July 30, 2007.

15. Stewart WF, Lipton RB, Celentano DD, et al. Prevalence of migraine headache in the United States. Relation to age, income, race, and other sociodemographic factors. *JAMA* 1992;267:64–9.

16. Lipton RB, Bigal ME, Diamond M, et al. for the AMPP Advisory Group. Migraine prevalence, disease burden, and the need for preventive therapy. *Neurology* 2007;68:343–9.

17. Goadsby PJ. Recent advances in the diagnosis and management of migraine. *BMJ* 2006;332:25–9.

18. Kaniecki R, Lucas S. Treatment of primary headache: preventive treatment of migraine. In: *Standards of Care for Headache Diagnosis and Treatment*. Chicago: National Headache Foundation, 2004:40–52.

19. Ramadan NM, Silberstein SD, Freitag FG, et al. for the US Headache Consortium. *Evidence-Based Guidelines for Migraine Headache in the Primary Care Setting: Pharmacological Management for Prevention of Migraine*. Available from: www.aan.com/professionals/practice/pdfs/gl0090.pdf. Accessed July 30, 2007.

20. Newman LC, Goadsby P, Lipton RB. Cluster and related headaches. *Med Clin North Am* 2001;85:997–1016.

21. Manzoni GC. Gender ratio of cluster headache over the years: a possible role of changes in lifestyle. *Cephalalgia* 1998;18:138–42.

22. Clusterheadaches.com. *Medical Information About Cluster Headaches*. Available from: www.clusterheadaches.com/about.html. Accessed July 30, 2007.

23. Beck E, Sieber WJ, Trejo R. Management of cluster headache. *Am Fam Physician* 2005;71:717–24.

10 • Fibromyalgia

Fibromyalgia is a common rheumatologic disorder. It has only been recognized in recent decades, and its pathogenesis is still not fully understood.

Fibromyalgia is characterized by chronic and widespread musculoskeletal aches, pain, and stiffness, soft tissue tenderness, general fatigue, sleep disturbances, and an increased incidence of depression, psychological distress, and autonomic dysfunction. The most common sites of pain include the neck, back, shoulders, pelvic girdle, and hands, but any part of the body can be affected [1].

Prevalence

Fibromyalgia has been well reported in the US, but racial and social dispositions have not been fully addressed.

* Overall prevalence has been estimated at 3% for women and 0.5% for men [2].
* Women are most often affected, representing 80–90% of fibromyalgia sufferers [3].
* Fibromyalgia can develop at any age, but most patients are in their 40s and 50s. It is rarely reported in children [3].
* There is some evidence of a genetic predisposition, but no clear pattern has yet been demonstrated [4].

- Fibromyalgia is the second most common disorder that rheumatologists encounter, and it has been calculated that one in every 10 patients evaluated in a medical practice may have fibromyalgia [5].

Patients often have comorbidities. Compared with people without fibromyalgia, fibromyalgia patients have been found to be significantly more likely to have painful neuropathies (23% vs 3% for comparison group), anxiety (5% vs 1%), and depression (12% vs 3%); they are also more likely to have used pain-related pharmacotherapy (65% vs 34%) [6].

> Fibromyalgia is the second most common disorder encountered by rheumatologists, where one in every 10 patients evaluated in a medical practice may be affected [5].

Pathogenesis

The cause of fibromyalgia is not yet established, but the most consistent research findings include the following:

- Substance P and nerve growth factor levels in the cerebrospinal fluid are elevated [7]. The increase in substance P has been related to exaggerated nociception, ie, increased pain sensitivity.
- Non-rapid eye movement (REM) sleep is disturbed by intrusions of dysfunctional alpha sleep patterns [8]. This correlates with patient reports of waking repeatedly and being unrefreshed by sleep (see **Chapter 18**) [5,9].

These and other findings have not thus far been linked by a unifying hypothesis. One researcher has described the syndrome as essentially one of diffuse hypersensitivity to pain (see **Box 1**).

Box 1. A 'sensory volume' problem?

Fibromyalgia may be a diffuse disorder of sensory volume control that alters the patient's threshold to pain and other stimuli, such as heat, noise, and strong odors. This hypersensitivity may result from neurobiological changes that affect the perception of nociceptive pain; these may be related to psychological factors [10].

Symptom	Description
Pain	Chronic and widespread, migrating to all parts of the body
	Variously described as aching, throbbing, stabbing, and shooting (patients often say that they "ache all over")
	May be associated with numbness and tingling
	May be aggravated by cold/humid weather, disturbed sleep, fatigue, and psychological and physiological stress
Fatigue	Not just tiredness, but severe exhaustion that interferes with the most simple of daily activities
	Patients sometimes feel as if every drop of energy has been drained from their body
Sleep problems	Sleep is regularly disrupted, and patients wake feeling tired and unrefreshed, presumably because of missing out on the restorative stage of sleep (see main text and **Chapter 18**)
	Sleep difficulties may be compounded by nighttime muscle spasms or restless legs syndrome
Other symptoms	These may include irritable bowel and bladder, headache and migraine, impaired memory and concentration, skin sensitivity and rashes, anxiety, depression, visual problems, or impaired concentration

Table 1. Symptoms of fibromyalgia [1–4].

Clinical presentation

Patients typically suffer from the symptoms of fibromyalgia for months or years before consulting a physician. The most characteristic and prevalent symptom is of widespread pain (see **Table 1**) [1,11].

Diagnosis

The American College of Rheumatology has set out criteria for the diagnosis of fibromyalgia [12]. The full criteria, which can be found at www.nfra.net, have two principal components:

- The presence of pain in all four quadrants of the body, as well as in the axial skeleton, for at least 3 months. The pain is often described as widespread or global.
- The presence of at least 11 of 18 anatomically specific tender points across the body. A tender point should hurt when a digital palpation pressure of 4 kg is applied. This is approximately the degree of pressure that would cause the skin under the examiner's nail to blanch.

Some clinicians consider these criteria over-rigid, and believe that fibromyalgia can be diagnosed based on the history and a smaller number of tender points [3].

Management

As in other pain syndromes, effective management consists of a combination of pharmacologic, psychological, and social supportive measures (see **Table 2**) [1–4,13–18]. An overriding principle is that, since the symptoms of fibromyalgia are so variable, treatment must be tailored to individual needs.

In June 2007, pregabalin capsules became the first drug to be approved by the Food and Drug Administration (FDA) specifically for the treatment of fibromyalgia [19]. The drug should be started at 75 mg twice daily PO, and may be increased to 150 mg twice daily within 1 week. The maximum dose is 450 mg/day; the dose should be adjusted for patients with reduced renal function [20].

> Pregabalin is the first drug to be approved by the FDA specifically for the treatment of fibromyalgia.

Treatment	Description
Cognitive measures: support, explanation, motivation	A professional and empathic approach combined with simple explanation and reassurance, ideally involving family members, is frequently helpful
	Fibromyalgia support groups can provide education and assistance
NSAIDs	NSAIDs and other analgesics are generally not effective
Opioids	Chronic opioid therapy is reserved for patients with severe pain and/or functional impairment who are not responsive to standard treatment measures
Antidepressants	TCAs may be effective
	The TCA dose is generally lower than that required to treat depression and tolerance may be poor; the medication should be instituted at a low dose and increased gradually, with regular monitoring
Gabapentinoids	Pregabalin has been shown to be efficacious, improving pain, sleep, and fatigue compared with placebo
	Pregabalin is well tolerated and can improve global measures and health-related quality of life
	In June 2007, pregabalin capsules became FDA-approved for the treatment of fibromyalgia
Psychological treatment	CBT and packages that include multimodal management with CBT, exercise, and support groups are effective
Other treatments	Fibromyalgia patients have benefited from acupuncture, exercise programs, massage, yoga, relaxation techniques, and breathing exercises
	It is often a question of what is readily available, combined with individual preference and response

Table 2. Management of fibromyalgia [1–4,13–18]. Specific treatments are addressed in more detail in later chapters. CBT: cognitive behavioral therapy; FDA: Food and Drug Administration; NSAID: nonsteroidal anti-inflammatory drug; TCA: tricyclic antidepressant.

References

1. National Fibromyalgia Association (NFA). *Fibromyalgia*. Available from: http://fmaware.org. Accessed July 30, 2007.
2. Goldenberg DL. Fibromyalgia syndrome a decade later: what have we learned? *Arch Intern Med* 1999;159:777–85.
3. Mayo Clinic. *Fibromyalgia*. Available from: www.mayoclinic.com. Accessed July 30, 2007.
4. Olson J. *Mapping Genes for Fibromyalgia. NIAMS Spotlight on Research. Fibromyalgia: Summaries of Research*, 2004. Available from: www.niams.nih.gov. Accessed July 30, 2007.
5. Gilliland RP. Fibromyalgia. *eMedicine*. Available from: www.emedicine.com/pmr/topic47.htm. Accessed July 30, 2007.

6. Berger A, Dukes E, Martin S, et al. Characteristics and healthcare costs of patients with fibromyalgia syndrome. *Int J Clin Pract* 2007;61:1498–508.

7. Russell IJ, Orr MD, Littman B, et al. Elevated cerebrospinal fluid levels of substance P in patients with the fibromyalgia syndrome. *Arthritis Rheum* 1994;37:1593–601.

8. Moldofsky H. Sleep and fibrositis syndrome. *Rheum Dis Clin North Am* 1989;15:91–103.

9. Crofford LJ. Neuroendocrine aspects of fibromyalgia. *J Musculoskeletal Pain* 1994;2:125–33.

10. Clauw DJ. Fibromyalgia: more than just a musculoskeletal disease. *Am Fam Physician* 1995;52:843–51.

11. Doherty M, Jones A. ABC of rheumatology. Fibromyalgia syndrome. *BMJ* 1995;310:386–9.

12. Wolfe F, Smythe HA, Yunus MB, et al. The American College of Rheumatology 1990 Criteria for the Classification of Fibromyalgia. Report of the Multicenter Criteria Committee. *Arthritis Rheum* 1990;33:160–72.

13. Goldenberg D, Mayskiy M, Mossey C, et al. A randomized, double-blind crossover trial of fluoxetine and amitriptyline in the treatment of fibromyalgia. *Arthritis Rheum* 1996;39:1852–9.

14. Anderberg UM, Marteinsdottir I, von Knorring L. Citalopram in patients with fibromyalgia – a randomized, double-blind, placebo-controlled study. *Eur J Pain* 2000;4:27–35.

15. Crofford LJ, Rowbotham MC, Mease PJ, et al. Pregabalin for the treatment of fibromyalgia syndrome: results of a randomized, double-blind, placebo-controlled trial. *Arthritis Rheum* 2005;52:1264–73.

16. Tofferi JK, Jackson JL, O'Malley PG. Treatment of fibromyalgia with cyclobenzaprine: a meta-analysis. *Arthritis Rheum* 2004;51:9–13.

17. Singh BB, Berman BM, Hadhazy VA, et al. A pilot study of cognitive behavioral therapy in fibromyalgia. *Altern Ther Health Med* 1998;4:67–70.

18. Keel PJ, Bodoky C, Gerhard U, et al. Comparison of integrated group therapy and group relaxation training for fibromyalgia. *Clin J Pain* 1998;14:232–8.

19. Food and Drug Administration (FDA). *FDA Approves First Drug for Treating Fibromyalgia*. Press release: June 21, 2007.

20. *Lyrica (Pregabalin): Prescribing Information*. Pfizer: June, 2007. Available from www.lyrica.com. Accessed July 30, 2007.

11 • Cancer pain

The National Cancer Institute's Surveillance Epidemiology and End Results Cancer Statistics Review estimates that in the USA 1,444,920 people will be diagnosed with and 559,650 people will die of cancer in 2007 [1]. Pain is one of the most common symptoms associated with cancer [2]. It often leads the individual to seek medical advice and, subsequently, to the detection of cancer. Furthermore, approximately 50% of all patients diagnosed with cancer and 80% with progressive disease will be in need of physician-prescribed analgesia [3]. Cancer pain is a composite entity (see the causes of pain, below) and efficient management, particularly in a palliative care setting, often requires a multimodal approach.

> "[Cancer pain is] a mosaic composed of acute pain, chronic pain, tumor-specific pain, and treatment-related pain cemented together by ongoing psychological responses of distress and suffering" [4].

Causes of pain

Pain in the cancer patient may be related to [2]:

- the tumor (eg, progression of the cancer)
- the treatment (eg, diagnostic or therapeutic procedures) – otherwise known as procedural pain
- causes unrelated to the cancer or the treatment

Assessment of pain
Initiation of analgesic therapy
Monitoring of analgesic efficacy
Management of adverse effects (eg, nausea, obstipation, sedation, itch)
Coordination between oncologist and patient

Table 1. Competence areas in the management of cancer pain.

Cancer-related pain can be caused by compression of visceral structures (eg, intestines, bile duct, ureter), invasion of neural structures (eg, plexopathy in Pancoast syndrome), cerebral metastases, osteolytic metastases, or skin ulcerations (eg, in vulvar cancer).

The most common *procedural pain* in cancer patients is probably postoperative pain following surgery. However, pleural taps, spinal taps, blood marrow sampling, and insertion of central venous catheters are all potential painful procedures.

During the last decade, more aggressive oncologic therapies have been introduced that have successfully increased the life expectancy and survival rate in patients with a number of malignancies [5]. However, these therapies may inadvertently increase the number of patients with chronic pain problems either due to the increased survival rate *per se* or due to sequelae following surgery (eg, postmastectomy syndrome, phantom pain), radiotherapy (eg, radiation-induced colitis), or chemotherapy (eg, painful polyneuropathy). Survivorship issues also include long-term posttraumatic psychosocial distress with depression and anxiety.

The physician should be able to initiate relevant analgesic therapy, and monitor analgesic efficacy and adverse effects (see **Table 1**). Cancer patients often present with a variety of symptoms in addition to pain, such as fatigue, nausea, insomnia, cachexia, constipation, shortness of breath, and anxiety. These symptoms may aggravate pain. On the other hand, pain and pain treatment can affect these symptoms, generating a vicious cycle. For example, constipation due to dehydration in a nauseated patient with an abdominal malignancy can lead to increased pain; if opioids are administered without additional laxatives, the patient will experience increased constipation and even more pain.

General treatment strategies

The effective management of pain in the cancer patient requires a combination of symptomatic and oncologic treatments. For example, a patient with primary breast cancer and painful osteolytic bone metastases is likely to receive immediate benefit from analgesic pharmacotherapy with an opioid and nonsteroidal anti-inflammatory drug (NSAID). Sustained pain relief with a combination of radiotherapy and bisphosphonates is often obtained following a delay of 2–3 weeks after the end of oncologic therapy.

The three-step analgesic ladder recommended by the World Health Organization since 1986 is a simple, esthetically attractive concept that has improved pharmacologic pain therapy [6]. Mild pain is treated with acetaminophen or an NSAID, while moderate or more intense pain may be treated with opioids. A pragmatic approach is recommended for severe pain. The first objective is to obtain pain relief during the night, the second to obtain relief during rest in the day, and the final, more difficult objective is to achieve pain relief during physical activity.

Evidence for analgesic polypharmacy

In the management of postoperative pain, a combination of morphine and NSAIDs, compared with morphine monotherapy, has been demonstrated to significantly increase analgesic efficacy, decrease opioid requirements, and decrease opioid-related adverse effects such as sedation and nausea [7,8]. The results have been less consistent in systematic reviews of cancer pain [4,9], although larger clinical studies seem to confirm a potential role for polypharmacy [10,11].

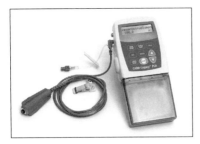

Figure 1. An electro-mechanical pump (Legacy, Deltec 6300), with patient-controlled device, for the parenteral administration of analgesics. The single-use drug reservoir is filled by the pharmacy.

With thanks to Per Rasmussen, Hvidovre University Hospital, Denmark.

The three-step analgesic ladder has some shortcomings:

- Neuropathic pain components, which are present in >50% of cancer patients with severe pain [12], do not readily respond to NSAIDs; adjuvant analgesics in combination with opioids are needed.
- Drugs for the management of adverse effects related to analgesic therapy (eg, constipation, nausea) should be given a prominent place in the ladder in order for the physician to avoid an inadvertent reduction in the patient's quality of life and in compliance.
- Finally, a number of patients will, at some point, need pain interventions, more specialized therapies such as patient-controlled analgesia with a pump for opioid administration (see **Figure 1**), or a spinal catheter for the administration of an opioid and a local anesthetic.

Figure 2 displays a more comprehensive analgesic ladder that takes these factors into account.

Pain assessment

The general principles of pain assessment are also applicable to the cancer patient with pain. An assessment should include questions targeted at 'where, how, and when' does the pain appear. Intensity scales such as the visual analog scale and the numeric rating scale are particularly helpful in monitoring treatment efficacy.

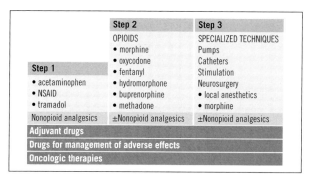

	Step 2	Step 3
	OPIOIDS	SPECIALIZED TECHNIQUES
	• morphine	Pumps
	• oxycodone	Catheters
Step 1	• fentanyl	Stimulation
• acetaminophen	• hydromorphone	Neurosurgery
• NSAID	• buprenorphine	• local anesthetics
• tramadol	• methadone	• morphine
Nonopioid analgesics	±Nonopioid analgesics	±Nonopioid analgesics
Adjuvant drugs		
Drugs for management of adverse effects		
Oncologic therapies		

Figure 2. A more comprehensive three-step analgesic ladder illustrating that the management of cancer-related pain is based upon oncologic therapies. Adjuvant drugs (drugs with primary indications other than analgesia) and drugs for the management of adverse effects (eg, laxatives, antiemetics) are important for patient compliance and successful analgesia. Step 3 includes advanced treatment (ie, specialized techniques from pumps for the parenteral administration of opioids to neurosurgical procedures). NSAID: nonsteroidal anti-inflammatory drug.

A pain diary may supply the physician with useful information; the patient should indicate pain intensity before and after medication, activity-related changes in pain intensity, diurnal variation in pain intensity, and the requirement for rescue medications. Benefits of using a pain diary include guidance for pain management behaviors and an enhanced sense of control for the patient. It is also a useful tool for communication [13].

Psychosocial and existential aspects of pain perception associated with the potential life-threatening disease must be considered and evaluated [14]. A number of relevant questionnaires for the assessment of depression and anxiety can serve as useful guides; the Edmonton Symptom Assessment System is a multidimensional instrument that can be used to evaluate symptoms in the cancer patient (see **Figure 3**) [15,16].

Neuropathic (cancer) pain states should be suspected when the following four classic criteria are seen:

- The pain area corresponds to the innervation territory of a nerve, nerve root (dermatome), or central nervous system structure.

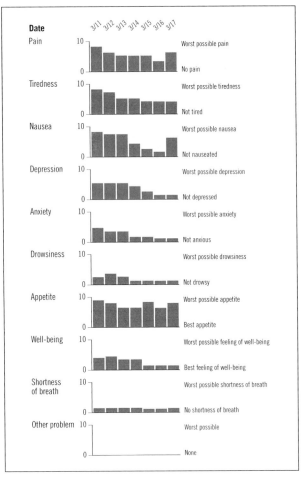

Figure 3. The Edmonton Symptom Assessment System scale (with example data shown).

Reproduced with permission from the American Medical Association (Bruera E, Kim HN. Cancer pain. *JAMA* 2003;290:2476–9).

- The pain is described as burning, tingling, pins and needles, electric, or stabbing [17].
- There are signs of sensory or motor dysfunction in the pain area (eg, allodynia, hyporeflexia) [17].

Pain syndrome	Cause
Cranial nerve neuralgia	Base of skull or leptomeningeal metastases, head and neck cancers
Mononeuropathy and other neuralgias	Rib metastases with intercostal nerve injury
Radiculopathy	Epidural mass, vertebral metastases, leptomeningeal metastases
Cervical plexopathy	Head and neck cancer with local extension, cervical lymph node metastases
Brachial plexopathy	Lymph node metastases from breast cancer or lymphoma, direct extension of Pancoast tumor
Lumbosacral plexopathy	Extension of colorectal cancer, cervical cancer, sarcoma, or lymphoma, breast cancer metastases
Paraneoplastic peripheral neuropathy	Small-cell lung cancer
Central pain	Spinal cord compression, cerebral metastases

Table 2. Clinical examples of neuropathic pain syndromes related to cancer and cancer therapies [18].

- Pain therapy has been unsuccessful with ordinary analgesics or the patient requires high doses of strong opioids. In addition, the pain is often perceived as distinctly abnormal and, frequently, is accentuated at night time.

Pain syndromes related to cancer and cancer therapies

Clinical examples of pain syndromes related to cancer and cancer therapies are listed in **Table 2** [17]. Sequelae to therapeutic interventions are listed in **Table 3** [17,19].

Neuropathic pain

Analgesic algorithm
Pharmacologic interventions
On a compassionate basis, according to the patient's clinical condition and pain mechanism, the physician may consider an empiric trial of one or more of the emergent topical, oral, or parenteral/intrathecal therapies [18].

Intervention	Sequelae
Extremely high doses of opioids or compromised opioid elimination	Widespread hyperalgesia
Postsurgical pain	Postmastectomy pain, postthoracotomy pain, phantom pain postamputation
Radiation therapy	Myelopathy, plexopathy, neuropathy
Chemotherapy	Neuropathy from cis-platinum, taxoids, vincristine
Corticosteroids	Perineal burning sensation, proximal myopathy
Intrathecal methotrexate	Acute meningitic syndrome

Table 3. Sequelae to therapeutic interventions [18,19].

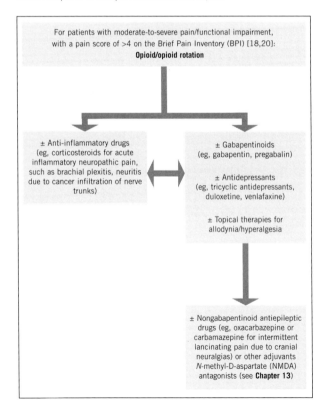

Procedures

The following are options for severe neuropathic pain due to cancer or sequelae of cancer treatment that are not amenable to conventional drug delivery routes [18]:

- implantable intrathecal pump or tunneled intraspinal catheter system for neuraxial analgesia (opioids ± bupivacaine, clonidine, or ziconotide)
- neurostimulatory procedures (spinal cord or motor cortex stimulation), largely for neuropathic pain as a sequela of cancer treatment
- neuroablative procedures (eg, dorsal root entry zone lesion, midline myelotomy)

Cancer-related bone pain states

Metastasis to bone is the most common cause of pain in cancer patients [21]. Bone pain is usually associated with direct tumor invasion of the bone, and is often severe and debilitating. Tumors that metastasize to bone most commonly originate in the breast, lung, prostate, or ovaries [22]. Multiple myeloma also causes painful bone lesions. More than two-thirds of patients with radiographically detectable lesions will experience bone pain, although many patients experience pain even before skeletal metastases become radiographically apparent.

Pain is often the presenting symptom of bone metastases, and the presence of focal pain in a cancer patient should trigger an investigation. Patients may experience a deep, powerful, throbbing pain punctuated by a sharper intense pain, often triggered by movement (incident or breakthrough pain; see **Chapter 12**). On examination, there might also be focal tenderness and swelling at the affected sites. Range of motion is usually severely limited, particularly if the joint space is involved. In many patients, normal activities such as deep breathing, coughing, or moving an affected limb can cause intense, often unbearable, pain.

The pain can be localized or referred to various sites. Bone pain due to metastases must be differentiated from other bone pain syndromes that are caused by nonneoplastic conditions, such as osteoarthritis, osteoporotic fractures, and osteomalacia.

Mechanisms of bone pain

Immunohistochemical studies have revealed an extensive network of nerve fibers in the vicinity of and within the skeleton. These are not only in the periosteum, but also in the cortical and trabecular bone, as well as in the bone marrow. Thinly myelinated and unmyelinated peptidergic sensory fibers, as well as sympathetic fibers, occur throughout the bone marrow, mineralized bone, and periosteum.

In recent animal models of cancer-related bone pain, nerve growth factor (NGF) has been shown to modulate inflammatory neuropathic pain states [23]. Anti-NGF therapy also has been shown to produce a significant reduction in both ongoing and movement-related pain behavior in animal models. This treatment has been found to be more effective than morphine [23,24].

It is believed that skeletal lesions result, at least in part, from a disruption of the normal balance between bone formation and bone resorption [25]. In the process, bone nociceptors respond to changes in the bone marrow, as well as cortical, trabecular, and periosteum microenvironments. Inflammatory, immunologic, and neuropathic mechanisms develop in the bone in response to the cancer insult, and the patient experiences pain. As osteolysis continues, bone integrity declines and patients become vulnerable to other complications, including pathologic fractures, nerve compression syndromes, spinal instability, and hypercalcemia.

Analgesic algorithm
Pharmacologic interventions

For patients with moderate to severe pain/functional impairment, with a pain score of >4 on the BPI [18]:

Opioid/opioid rotation + IV bisphosphonate
(eg, pamidronate, zoledronic acid, ibandronate)

± Anti-inflammatory drugs (eg, corticosteroids, NSAIDs)

± Gabapentinoids, antidepressants, mexiletine,
N-methyl-D-aspartate antagonists

Procedures

The following are options for severe pain/functional impairment or treatment that is not amenable to conventional drug delivery routes [18]:

- implantable intrathecal pump or tunneled intraspinal catheter system for neuraxial analgesia (opioids ± bupivacaine, clonidine, or ziconotide)
- radiation or radiopharmaceutical therapy
- palliative surgery (vertebroplasty, kyphoplasty) for large lytic lesions with risk of fracture
- neuroablative procedures

Visceral pain

Visceral pain is common in patients with cancer. It becomes evident during cancer infiltration, compression, distension, or stretching of thoracic and/or abdominal viscera. It can be either an early or late manifestation of cancer. Visceral nociceptors are activated by noxious stimuli, including inflammation of the mucosa and omentum and stretching of hollow viscera, as well as the organ capsule. Visceral pain is generally diffuse and caused by obstructive syndromes due to tumor involvement of the organ or the organ capsule. Pain can be caused by a primary tumor or metastatic disease to an organ [18].

Visceral pain is often described as dull, squeezing, colicky, sharp, and deep aching. It can be intermittent or continuous, and is often perceived as generalized lassitude. Visceral pain is poorly localized and can be accompanied by other symptoms such as nausea, fatigue, and diaphoresis. It is frequently referred to cutaneous areas overlying or adjacent to the affected structure; referral patterns can vary, and can even be distant from the underlying malignancy (eg, an aching and gnawing right shoulder pain that indicates the presence of hepatic metastases or diaphragmatic irritation; pancreatic and endometrial cancers can manifest as back pain; prostate cancer pain can appear in the abdomen or lower extremities). The clinician must be knowledgeable about pain referral patterns in order to treat the syndrome with precision [18].

Types of visceral cancer pain
Hepatic capsular pain
Hepatic capsular pain can occur with a primary hepatocellular carcinoma or, more commonly, with liver metastases. The inflammation caused by the disease can result in capsular stretching and produce pain, which is dull and aching, in the right subcostal region. Movement might exacerbate the pain; deep breaths cause right diaphragmatic irritation. The treatment for this syndrome is analgesic doses of corticosteroids, given in divided doses, and opioid analgesics.

Retroperitoneal pain syndrome
Retroperitoneal pain syndrome is most common in pancreatic cancer and retroperitoneal lymphadenopathy. The pain is exacerbated by recumbency and alleviated by forward flexion. The pain is dull, diffuse, and poorly localized. This type of pain should be differentiated from epidural metastasis. A careful examination and appropriate imaging can confirm the diagnosis.

Intestinal obstruction
Intestinal obstruction can be the result of a gastrointestinal tumor, adhesions, or intra-abdominal or pelvic space-occupying lesions. The pain is characterized as colicky. It is usually associated with nausea and/or vomiting, anorexia, and bloating. Another cause of this syndrome can be an atonic

140

bowel due to ischemia, autonomic denervation, or primary cancer therapies (including radiotherapy).

Mechanisms of pain

Visceral carcinomatosis can cause pain via a number of mechanisms, including peritoneal inflammation, malignant adhesions, and ascites. Tense ascites produce discomfort from abdominal wall stretching, and can manifest as low back pain. Pelvic and perineal pain can occur in malignancies that arise in the pelvis, including colorectal and genitourinary tumors. The tumor invades the pelvic floor and frequently causes both nociceptive and neuropathic pain. Occasionally, patients experience painful spasms in the rectum, bladder, or urethra. The visceral component of this pain syndrome can be marked by tenesmus.

Analgesic algorithm

Pharmacologic interventions

For patients with moderate to severe pain/functional impairment, with a pain score of >4 on the BPI [18]:

Opioid/opioid rotation ± anticholinergic agents

Corticosteroids, octreotide

± Gabapentinoids, antidepressants

Procedures

The following are options for severe pain/functional impairment or treatment that is not amenable to conventional drug delivery routes [18]:

- implantable intrathecal pump or tunneled intraspinal catheter system for neuraxial analgesia (opioids ± bupivacaine, clonidine, or ziconotide)
- palliative surgery (eg, colostomies, if clinically indicated)

- neurolytic blocks (eg, celiac plexus, superior hypogastric plexus, ganglion impar, epidural neurolysis)
- neuroablative procedures

Case study: treatment of neuropathic cancer pain with antidepressants and anticonvulsants[a]

A 68-year-old woman with a history of metastatic breast cancer presented with 4 months of progressive pain in her right shoulder, arm, and lateral hand. There was known metastatic disease to bone and the mediastinal lymph nodes. About 1 year ago, she developed discomfort in the right side of her neck and subsequently underwent radiotherapy to control enlarging right supraclavicular adenopathy. She had experienced no pain at this site until the current pain began. For the past 6 months she had been receiving chemotherapy with paclitaxel, and the disease in the bone and mediastinum appeared to be stable. She had difficulty sleeping, said she was depressed, and had difficulty in carrying out her usual daily activities.

She had been taking controlled-release morphine for some time and using short-acting morphine for breakthrough pain (see **Chapter 12** for detailed information on breakthrough pain). Her use of the short-acting drug had increased to 4–6 times daily in the past 2 months. The supplemental dose of morphine did not provide relief.

A computed tomography (CT) scan showed a discrete mass in the supraclavicular region and several nodules in the superior right lung. Comparison to an earlier CT scan confirmed that the masses were new, and consistent with malignant brachial plexopathy.

New chemotherapy was instituted, and treatment of the neuropathic pain began with further escalation of the morphine dose. However, the increase yielded only a slight benefit and with some increase in mental clouding. Given the patient's

[a]Abridged with permission from Biolink Communications (McDonald AA, Portenoy RK. How to use antidepressants and anticonvulsants as adjuvant analgesics in the treatment of neuropathic cancer pain. *J Support Oncol* 2006;4:43–52).

insomnia and depressed mood, a trial of desipramine was instituted, increasing to 100 mg at night. The patient reported better sleep and a modest improvement in pain, but some increase in morning fatigue. Treatment with gabapentin was added, and over 2 weeks was gradually increased to 1,800 mg twice daily. The patient reported a significant reduction in pain. Sleep had normalized, and her mood was significantly better. She described the pain as constant, but "never intolerable".

Summary

Advances are being made in our comprehension of the various mechanisms underlying neuropathic, bone, and visceral pain. If a patient presents with a difficult cancer pain syndrome, a comprehensive pain assessment and aggressive intervention are needed. Therapeutic interventions can be employed in an escalating regimen to counteract the intensity and the disabling nature of the patient's difficult cancer pain syndrome. The employment of agents from a variety of pharmacologic classes represents a contemporary standard approach to pain management. At present, the management of the difficult cancer pain syndrome calls for a balanced combination of therapies that will include analgesic medications, adjuvants, and oncologic, anesthesiologic, or surgical procedures.

References

1. Ries LAG, Melbert D, Krapcho M, et al., Editors. *SEER Cancer Statistics Review, 1975 2004*. Bethesda: National Cancer Institute. Available from: http://seer.cancer.gov/statfacts/html/all.html. Accessed October 12, 2007.
2. National Comprehensive Cancer Network (NCCN). *NCCN Clinical Practice Guidelines in Oncology: Adult Cancer Pain*. NCCN, 2007.
3. Bruera E, Kim HN. Cancer pain. *JAMA* 2003;290:2476–9.
4. Carr DB, Goudas LC, Balk EM, et al. Evidence report on the treatment of pain in cancer patients. *J Natl Cancer Inst Monogr* 2004;32:23–31.
5. Stewart BW, Kleihues P, Editors. *World Cancer Report*. Lyon, France: WHO International Agency for Research on Cancer, 2003.
6. Reid C, Davies A. The World Health Organization three-step analgesic ladder comes of age. *Palliat Med* 2004;18:175–6.
7. Elia N, Lysakowski C, Tramer MR. Does multimodal analgesia with acetaminophen, nonsteroidal antiinflammatory drugs, or selective cyclooxygenase-2 inhibitors and patient-controlled analgesia morphine offer advantages over morphine alone? Metaanalyses of randomized trials. *Anesthesiology* 2005;103:1296–304.

8. Marret E, Kurdi O, Zufferey P, et al. Effects of nonsteroidal antiinflammatory drugs on patient-controlled analgesia morphine side effects: meta-analysis of randomized controlled trials. *Anesthesiology* 2005;102:1249–60.

9. McNicol E, Strassels SA, Goudas L, et al. NSAIDs or paracetamol, alone or combined with opioids, for cancer pain. *Cochrane Database Syst Rev* 2005;(1):CD005180.

10. Mercadante S, Fulfaro F, Casuccio A. A randomised controlled study on the use of anti-inflammatory drugs in patients with cancer pain on morphine therapy: effects on dose-escalation and a pharmacoeconomic analysis. *Eur J Cancer* 2002;38:1358–63.

11. Caraceni A, Zecca E, Bonezzi C, et al. Gabapentin for neuropathic cancer pain: a randomized controlled trial from the Gabapentin Cancer Pain Study Group. *J Clin Oncol* 2004;22:2909–17.

12. Portenoy RK, Payne D, Jacobsen P. Breakthrough pain: characteristics and impact in patients with cancer pain. *Pain* 1999;81:129–34.

13. National Cancer Institute. *Pain Assessment*. National Institutes of Health. Available from: www.cancer.gov. Accessed August 30, 2007.

14. Otis-Green S, Sherman R, Perez M, et al. An integrated psychosocial-spiritual model for cancer pain management. *Cancer Pract* 2002;10(Suppl. 1):S58–65.

15. *Guidelines for using the Edmonton Symptom Assessment System (ESAS)*. Available from: www.palliative.org. Accessed August 30, 2007.

16. Bruera E, Schoeller T, Wenk R, et al. A prospective multicenter assessment of the Edmonton staging system for cancer pain. *J Pain Symptom Manage* 1995;10:348–55.

17. Paice JA. Mechanisms and management of neuropathic pain in cancer. *J Support Oncol* 2003;1:107–20.

18. Pappagallo M, Shaiova L, Perlov E, et al. Difficult pain syndromes: bone pain, visceral pain, neuropathic pain. In: Berger AM, Shuster JL, Von Roenn JH, Editors. *Principles and Practice of Palliative Care and Supportive Oncology*, 3rd Edn. Philadelphia: Lippincott Williams & Wilkins, 2006.

19. Angst MS, Clark JD. Opioid-induced hyperalgesia: a qualitative systematic review. *Anesthesiology* 2006;104:570–87.

20. Cleeland CS, Ryan KM. Pain assessment: global use of the Brief Pain Inventory. *Ann Acad Med Singapore* 1994;23:129–38.

21. Portenoy RK, Kanner R, Foley KM. *Pain Syndromes With Cancer*. Philadelphia: WB Saunders, 1996:191–215.

22. Mercadante S. Malignant bone pain: pathophysiology and treatment. *Pain* 1997;69:1–18.

23. Sevcik MA, Ghilardi JR, Peters CM, et al. Anti-NGF therapy profoundly reduces bone cancer pain and the accompanying increase in markers of peripheral and central sensitization. *Pain* 2005;115:128–41.

24. Halvorson KG, Kubota K, Sevcik MA, et al. A blocking antibody to nerve growth factor attenuates skeletal pain induced by prostate tumor cells growing in bone. *Cancer Res* 2005;65:9426–35.

25. Lipton A. Pathophysiology of bone metastases: how this knowledge may lead to therapeutic intervention. *J Support Oncol* 2004;2:205–23.

12 • Breakthrough pain

Definition and prevalence

Breakthrough pain (BTP) has been defined as a transitory worsening of pain or an exacerbation of pain that occurs on a stable background or baseline pattern of a chronic pain condition in an opioid-tolerant patient. The chronic pain condition may be either cancer- or noncancer-related in origin (eg, arthritis, low back pain, diabetic neuropathy) [1,2].

The characteristics and epidemiology of BTP in cancer pain have been extensively evaluated. The majority of patients with cancer pain (64.8% of patients in one study) are known to suffer from BTP [3].

In contrast, noncancer pain-related BTP has not yet been thoroughly studied. A 2001 survey of 43 patients with noncancer pain conditions indicated a prevalence of BTP in >50% of patients [4]. A more recent survey of 228 patients with chronic noncancer pain showed a high prevalence of BTP; in particular, 52% of patients with low back pain reported daily BTP. The median daily number of BTP episodes in these patients was two (range 0–12) and the average duration was 60 minutes. In the vast majority of cases, BTP was related to activity [5].

BTP and poor medical outcome

Several studies have indicated that the presence of clinically significant BTP is associated with higher patient morbidity, decreased level of function, worsening of quality of life, and increased depression. Patients with clinically significant or poorly controlled BTP have reported worse treatment satisfaction and higher healthcare utilization (eg, emergency department visits and hospitalizations) when compared with patients who have no BTP or well-controlled BTP [3,6–8].

Assessment

The physician should ensure that persistent pain is adequately controlled before assessing for BTP. Besides brief questionnaires (eg, the BTP questionnaire – see **Table 1**), pain diaries can be used to assess persistent pain characteristics and BTP, and to obtain more comprehensive patient information. A pain diary is a reliable tool for gathering over time the relevant BTP characteristics, such as occurrence and nature, predictability, frequency, duration, time to peak severity, intensity, interference with activities, and response to treatment. The diary is useful both at the initial patient evaluation and at follow-up visits. **Figure 1** shows a sample of a completed pain diary, developed by the American Pain Foundation. A blank copy of a pain diary is available at the Foundation's website (www.painfoundation.org).

Following the initiation of fast-acting or immediate-release opioids for BTP, each patient needs to be carefully assessed. In order to do this, the 'four A' guidelines should be followed [9]. The 'four A' guidelines are intended to help clinicians to assess and document their observations when treating chronic pain patients who are on opioid therapy. They are based on the assumption that systematic pain assessment and documentation can assist in improving patient care, providing a rationale for treatment decisions, and establishing the type of

Occurrence and nature
1. Do you have attacks of intense pain, also called BTP, that are superimposed to your baseline chronic pain? If yes, please proceed with the following questions.
2. Does the pain in your BTP attacks have similar or different characteristics when compared with your baseline chronic pain?

Predictability, precipitated by event
3. Does movement or a specific activity trigger your BTP, or is your BTP spontaneous, not evoked by any activity, or does it occur just before you take your next dose of pain medication?

Frequency, number of episodes per day
4. On average, how many attacks do you have a day?

Duration
5. How long does each attack last?

Time to peak severity
6. How long does it take to pick up to its maximum intensity?

Severity
7. On average, what number would you use to rate your attacks on a scale of 0–10, with 0 being no pain and 10 being the worst pain you can imagine?

Quality of life
8. Do your BTP attacks interfere with your daily activities at home or at work? Do you feel that your mood and quality of life would be better without BTP?
9. How is your sleep? Does the BTP wake you up at night? Does your BTP make it difficult for you to fall asleep?

Treatment
10. Are the medications you have used for BTP effective? How long does the pain medication take to work, and what percentage of pain relief do you get from the medication? How long does the relief last?

Table 1. The breakthrough pain (BTP) assessment questionnaire.

careful medical practice expected by the regulatory community [9]. The four *A*s are:

1. *A*nalgesia
2. *A*ctivities of daily living
3. *A*dverse events
4. *A*berrant drug-related behaviors

Risk management in opioid therapy is discussed in more detail in **Chapter 15**.

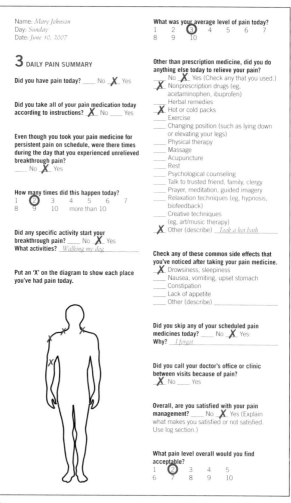

Figure 1. The 'daily pain summary' aspect of a pain diary. Steps 1 and 2 of the diary (not shown) are a daily pain chart and daily pain log, respectively. In these steps, the patient connects points on a graph to indicate their pain level throughout the day; lists their medications and time of dosing; and connects any nonmedicine therapy or activities/exercise to points on the graph. The patient may also add notes for and about visits with the healthcare provider, side effects from treatments that he/she is experiencing, and any problems that he/she is having coping with the pain.

Abbreviated with permission from the American Pain Foundation. (*Pain Notebook*. Available from: www.painfoundation.org.)

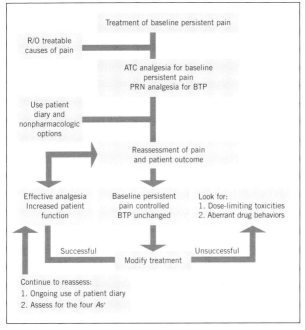

Figure 2. General approach to the management of breakthrough pain (BTP). ATC: around the clock; PRN: as needed; R/O: rule out. ªThe 'four As' are analgesia, activities of daily living, adverse events, and aberrant drug-related behavior.

Reproduced with permission from MediMedia USA (Bennett D, Burton AW, Fishman S, et al. Consensus panel recommendations for the assessment and management of breakthrough pain. Part 2: Management. *Pharm Ther* 2005;30:354–61).

Management

When available, primary and specific therapies should be used to treat the underlying disease that causes the pain. However, chronic pain, including BTP, often achieves a clinical status of disease on its own, requiring assessment, treatment prevention, and a complex management strategy (see **Figure 2**) [10]. Clinicians managing BTP should always consider, when appropriate, combinations of nonpharmacologic treatments (eg, physical therapy techniques – see **Chapter 17**) and pharmacologic treatments. The baseline pain needs to be treated successfully, often requiring around-the-clock doses of an

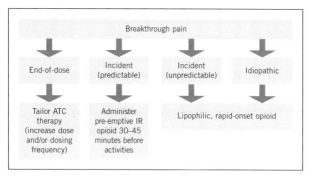

Figure 3. Management of breakthrough pain subtypes. ATC: around-the-clock; IR: immediate-release.

Reproduced with permission from Blackwell (McCarberg BH. The treatment of breakthrough pain. *Pain Med* 2007;8[Suppl. 1]:S8–13).

analgesic medication. Ideally, the medication for BTP should have a rapid onset of action and an adequate duration of analgesia to provide effective coverage of the BTP peak severity.

Management of BTP subtypes

Several BTP subtypes have been defined, each of which has different characteristics (see **Figure 3**) [10]. Through understanding these characteristics, the clinician can prescribe effective rescue medications.

'End-of-dose' BTP is defined as a BTP episode that occurs soon before the next scheduled dose of the patient's baseline pain medication [10]. These episodes can often be controlled by increasing the dose and/or shortening the dosing interval of the patient's baseline analgesia. However, the risk of adverse events may be increased [11].

Incident BTP is caused by activity, and is usually predictable. It may be treated with oral, short-acting opioids such as hydrocodone, hydromorphone, codeine, morphine, or oxycodone [10]. These have an onset of action of approximately 30 minutes; therefore, once the triggering activity has been identified, a short-acting oral opioid can be pre-emptively administered 30–45 minutes before the activity. The duration of effect is approximately 4 hours.

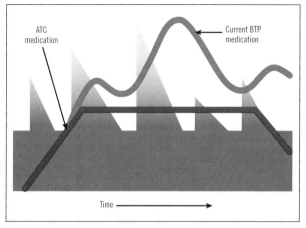

Figure 4. Common difficulties with around-the-clock (ATC) and breakthrough pain (BTP) treatment regimens. Peaks represent BTP that is poorly controlled by the ATC regimen prescribed for persistent baseline pain.

Unpredictable incident BTP and idiopathic BTP are more challenging to treat. The peak intensity of these subtypes usually occurs within 3–5 minutes following pain onset, and the episode generally lasts for approximately 30 minutes [11]. **Figure 4** shows the result of prescribing an oral, short-acting opioid: with an onset of action of 30 minutes, the drug comes into effect as the BTP event subsides. In other words, the onset and duration of action of the drug do not match the patient's pattern of pain.

In these cases, an analgesic with a more rapid onset of action is required. Preparations of transmucosal fentanyl have specific Food and Drug Administration indications for cancer-related BTP. Fentanyl is a lipophilic opioid. When given transmucosally, fentanyl can produce onset of analgesia within approximately 10–15 minutes postadministration [12–15], and has a duration of action of at least 2 hours [13]. Oral transmucosal fentanyl citrate has been reported to produce a greater analgesic effect, better global satisfaction, and a more rapid onset of action than oral, short-acting opioids or placebo [16]. It may provide a better 'fit' with the patient's pattern of pain (see **Figure 5**).

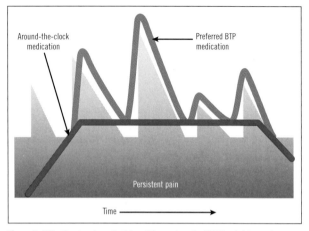

Figure 5. Effective treatment of breakthrough pain (BTP) might require an agent that provides rapid onset of analgesia (ie, within 10 minutes) and a duration of action sufficient to cover the duration of the BTP peak of intensity (ie, at least 1–2 hours).

Reproduced with permission from Cephalon, Inc.

Opioid analgesics are discussed in more detail in **Chapter 14**, and the risk management issues surrounding the use of opioids are detailed in **Chapter 15**.

References

1. Portenoy RK, Hagen NA. Breakthrough pain: definition, prevalence and characteristics. *Pain* 1990;41:273–81.

2. Bennett DS, Burton AW, Fishman S, et al. Consensus Panel Recommendations for the Assessment and Management of Breakthrough Pain. Part 1: Assessment. *Pharm Ther* 2005;30:296–301.

3. Caraceni A, Martini C, Zecca E, et al. Working Group of an IASP Task Force on Cancer Pain. Breakthrough pain characteristics and syndromes in patients with cancer pain. An international survey. *Palliative Med* 2004;18:177–83.

4. Zeppetella G, O'Doherty CA, Collins S. Prevalence and characteristics of breakthrough pain in patients with nonmalignant terminal disease admitted to a hospice. *Palliative Med* 2001;15:243–6.

5. Portenoy RK, Bennett DS, Rauck R, et al. Prevalence and characteristics of breakthrough pain in opioid-treated patients with chronic noncancer pain. *J Pain* 2006;7:583–91.

6. Portenoy RK, Payne D, Jacobsen P. Breakthrough pain: characteristics and impact in patients with cancer pain. *Pain* 1999;81:129–34.

7. Bruns D, Disorbio J, Bennett DS, et al. Degree of pain intolerance and adverse outcomes in chronic noncancer pain patients. *J Pain* 2005;6(Suppl.):S74(abstr.).

8.   Fortner BV, Okon TA, Portenoy RK. A survey of pain-related hospitalizations, emergency department visits, and physician office visits reported by cancer patients with and without history of breakthrough pain. *J Pain* 2002;3:38–44.

9.   National Pain Education Council. *Pain Assessment and Documentation Tool and Guidebook*. Available from: www.npecweb.org. Accessed August 30, 2007.

10. McCarberg BH. The treatment of breakthrough pain. *Pain Med* 2007;8(Suppl. 1):S8–13.

11. Bennett D, Burton AW, Fishman S, et al. Consensus panel recommendations for the assessment and management of breakthrough pain. Part 2: Management. *Pharm Ther* 2005;30:354–61.

12. Farrar JT, Cleary J, Rauck R, et al. Oral transmucosal fentanyl citrate: randomized, double-blinded, placebo-controlled trial for treatment of breakthrough pain in cancer patients. *J Natl Cancer Inst* 1998;90:611–16.

13. Portenoy RK, Taylor D, Messina J, et al. A randomized, placebo-controlled study of fentanyl buccal tablet for breakthrough pain in opioid-treated patients with cancer. *Clin J Pain* 2006:22:805–11.

14. Simpson DM, Messina J, Xie F, et al. Fentanyl buccal tablet for the relief of breakthrough pain in opioid-tolerant adult patients with chronic neuropathic pain: a multicenter, randomized, double-blind, placebo-controlled study. *Clin Ther* 2007;29:588–601.

15. Portenoy RK, Messina J, Xie F, et al. Fentanyl buccal tablet (FBT) for relief of breakthrough pain in opioid-treated patients with chronic low back pain: a randomized, placebo-controlled study. *Curr Med Res Opin* 2007;23:223–33.

16. Zeppetella G, Ribeiro MD. Opioids for the management of breakthrough (episodic) pain in cancer patients. *Cochrane Database Syst Rev* 2006;(1):CD004311.

13 • Nonopioid analgesics and adjuvants

Treatment with nonopioid analgesics represents the first step on the World Health Organization (WHO) analgesic ladder, which was first published in 1986. The WHO ladder was originally proposed for the treatment of cancer pain and has been widely influential [1]. Physicians should not, however, adhere too rigidly to the ladder model, as there are exceptions – in particular, severe, disabling pain should be immediately treated aggressively with a combination of agents, including opioids.

Nonselective, nonsteroidal anti-inflammatory drugs

Nonselective, nonsteroidal anti-inflammatory drugs (NNSAIDs or NSAIDs) (see **Table 1**) are thought to reduce inflammatory joint and skeletal-muscle pain. NSAIDs principally exert their effects by inhibiting the enzyme cyclooxygenase (COX), thus inhibiting prostaglandin $(PG)E_2$ synthesis. This results in both central and peripheral anti-inflammatory and analgesic effects [2,3].

A Cochrane review has found no evidence that any individual NSAID is better than any other for pain relief in low back pain [4]. Of note, a systematic review of 19 randomized controlled trials found no difference between NSAIDs and placebo for patients with sciatica [5].

Nonselective COX inhibitors	Selective COX-2 inhibitors
Aspirin, ibuprofen, indomethacin, ketoprofen, naproxen, piroxicam, sulindac, tolmetin	Celecoxib

Table 1. Some nonsteroidal anti-inflammatory drugs. COX: cyclooxygenase.

Indications and contraindications

- NSAIDs are indicated for the treatment of mild to moderate inflammatory or nonneuropathic pain [2].
- In postoperative pain, systematic reviews have demonstrated a higher analgesic efficacy for NSAIDs compared with acetaminophen [6–8].
- A Cochrane review found no clear evidence to support the superior safety or efficacy of one NSAID over another in cancer pain [9].
- There are a number of side effects of and contra-indications to the use of NSAIDs (see the next section); the choice of NSAID will depend on the risk of these side effects in an individual patient (eg, bleeding, history of gastric problems).
- If the pain is relatively severe, a reasonable first choice is an NSAID supplemented with opioids.
- Note that NSAIDs have opioid dose-sparing effects, and may reduce opioid-related side effects such as sedation and nausea [2].

Side effects

- All NSAIDs carry a risk of serious gastrointestinal (GI) complications: bleeding, perforation, and development of strictures [2]. Use with caution in patients at GI risk (see **Table 2**).
- Aspirin can cause gastric irritation after a single dose [10]. In common with other NSAIDs, it significantly increases bleeding time. NSAIDs should not be combined due to a dramatically increased risk of serious complications (the only exception is aspirin in antithrombotic doses: 75–125 mg).

History of ulcer disease and/or GI bleeding (10-fold increased risk for developing a GI bleed compared with patients with neither of these risk factors)
Concomitant use of oral corticosteroids or anticoagulants
Longer duration of NSAID therapy
Smoking
Use of alcohol
Older age
Poor general health status

Table 2. Patients at particular gastrointestinal (GI) risk with nonsteroidal anti-inflammatory drug (NSAID) use, as listed by the Food and Drug Administration NSAID labeling template, 2005.

- The risk of complications increases with the dose and duration of treatment [11].
- Chronic NSAID use increases the risk of renal insufficiency, particularly in patients with diabetes [12]; patients should be monitored for signs of reduced renal function (creatinine).
- Many patients with chronic pain take over-the-counter NSAIDs. The patient should be asked about all over-the-counter medicines in order to avoid inappropriate or excessive usage or adverse effects [13].

> Monitor all long-term NSAID use – ask about over-the-counter medications, particularly in patients at high risk of side effects.

COX-2 inhibitors

The substantial benefits of NSAIDs unfortunately come at a price: >2,000 people die each year as a result of NSAID-induced upper GI damage [14]. As many as 40% of serious GI complications following the administration of nonselective NSAIDs occur distal to the duodenum, in the small and large intestine [15].

The *COX-2 inhibitors* belong to a class of drugs that selectively inhibit COX-2, the enzyme involved in the inflammation

> **Box 1.** The current status of cyclooxygenase (COX)-2 inhibitors.
>
> In **September 2004**, the manufacturer of rofecoxib voluntarily withdrew the drug from the worldwide market due to a study that found an increased risk of developing a thrombotic event with rofecoxib compared with placebo.
>
> Seven months later, in **April 2005**, the Food and Drug Administration (FDA) recommended the withdrawal of valdecoxib from the market due to a risk of severe, life-threatening cutaneous reactions (erythema multiforme, Stevens–Johnson syndrome, toxic epidermal necrolysis).
>
> In **June 2005**, the FDA requested that the labeling for all NSAIDs, including celecoxib, show a black box warning highlighting the potential for an increased risk of cardiovascular (acute myocardial infarction) and cerebrovascular (stroke) events, and the serious, potentially life-threatening gastrointestinal bleeding associated with their use. See www.fda.gov/medwatch for more information.

pathway, while sparing the constitutive COX-1, thereby reducing GI toxicity. Several studies have provided evidence for a significant reduction in NSAID-induced gastroenteropathy with celecoxib compared with traditional NSAIDs [16,17].

Pivotal clinical trials from 2000 onwards indicated that COX-2 inhibitors are as effective as NSAIDs in reducing pain and improving function in rheumatoid arthritis and osteoarthritis [18,19]. However, the question of unwanted side effects – in particular, the risk of serious cardiovascular events – became the subject of international debate. The issues are summarized in references by Jones and Jüni et al. [14,20]. Celecoxib is currently the only COX-2 selective NSAID available (see **Box 1**) [21].

A 2006 meta-analysis (138 randomized controlled trials, n=145,373) reported that selective COX-2 inhibitor use was associated with a 42% relative increase in the incidence of serious vascular events (eg, myocardial infarction, stroke) [22]. Of note, with the exception of naproxen, several traditional NSAIDs were also associated with a similar excess risk of thrombotic events. In the light of these and other results, it is suggested that other pharmacologic and nonpharmacologic options need to be considered. These may be effective, safe, and even less costly [23].

"Rather than lamenting the loss of COX-2 inhibitors ... we will best serve our patients by thinking creatively about other approaches to their pain. Presenting a menu of possible treatments and working with patients to choose those that best suit their lifestyle and health beliefs is the optimal way to find solutions for their often chronic pain. Patients may not have to live with pain if they can live with the solutions that we explore with them" [23].

Acetaminophen

Acetaminophen has analgesic and antipyretic properties. However, it is still unclear how acetaminophen produces its analgesic action. Acetaminophen has been found to selectively suppress peripheral PGE_2 release, indirectly activate the cannabinoid 1 receptors, perhaps block a splice variant of COX-1 (called COX-1b or COX-3, primarily identified in canine brains), activate the central nervous system (CNS) serotoninergic pathway, and, lastly, downregulate proinflammatory interleukin (IL)-1β production [24, 25].

Research has indicated that pain relief with acetaminophen is very similar, milligram for milligram, to that with aspirin [26]. Although acetaminophen does not damage the gastric mucosa and has no platelet-aggregation toxicity, it can have chronic adverse renal or hepatic effects. A recent trial found that up to 44% of healthy patients who were randomized to 4 g/day of acetaminophen experienced serum alanine aminotransferase elevations greater than three times the upper normal limit, compared with no elevation with placebo [27]. Acetaminophen, alone or in combination, should therefore be restricted to not more than 2 g/day [2].

Acetaminophen should be avoided or used with caution in patients with liver impairment and those who are at risk of liver disease (eg, alcohol abusers), and in potentially suicidal patients [2]. *Overdose is a medical emergency.*

Acetaminophen may be the first choice for the treatment of mild chronic pain, or in combination with other agents in mild to moderate pain. It is generally well tolerated [2].

Analgesic adjuvants

An 'analgesic adjuvant' is a pharmacologic agent that usually has one or more treatment indications other than pain, and/or is added to a primary analgesic agent (eg, NSAID, opioid) in an attempt to potentiate improvements in the patient's pain and function.

Advances in molecular biology and neuroscience have generated attention in a variety of emerging analgesic adjuvants (see **Table 3**). The major rationale for introducing adjuvants is to improve the balance of efficacy and adverse effects. An adjuvant should be considered when [28]:

- the 'ceiling dose' (due to toxicity) of a primary analgesic has been reached
- the therapeutic benefit of a primary analgesic has plateaued (eg, true efficacy limit, tolerance)
- the primary analgesic is contraindicated (eg, substance abuse, aberrant behavior, organ failure, allergy)
- a variety of painful symptoms demands different medications for broader coverage
- a patient has disabling, nonpainful complaints such as insomnia, depression, anxiety, and fatigue

These all worsen the patient's quality of life and function. Indeed, the treatment outcome in pain management is both satisfactory pain relief *and* improvement in function.

Antiepilepsy drugs

Gabapentinoids

The gabapentinoid antiepilepsy drugs (AEDs), gabapentin and pregabalin, both have established efficacy for neuropathic pain [28]. Originally, gabapentin was chemically designed to resemble and act as the neurotransmitter γ-aminobutyric acid (GABA). However, subsequent studies have shown that gabapentin does not interact with either GABA-A or GABA-B receptors, that it is not metabolically converted into GABA or a GABA agonist, and that it does not block GABA reuptake or degradation. Moreover, the two gabapentinoids do not appear to have affinity for a number of other common receptor sites, with the exception of the $\alpha_2\delta$ subunit of the voltage-gated calcium channels. Therefore, the analgesic effect of gabapentin and pregabalin appears to be linked to modulation of the intracellular Ca^{2+} influx into nociceptive neurons via their binding to voltage-gated calcium channels – in particular, to the $\alpha_2\delta$ subunit of the channel [28].

Gabapentinoids are not metabolized and are essentially excreted in the urine as unchanged drugs. In order to prevent toxicity in patients with compromised renal function, the dosage of these medications needs to be carefully adjusted [29].

Gabapentin

Gabapentin has been regarded as the first-line treatment for neuropathic pain syndromes, probably because of its favorable toxicity profile and lack of major drug interactions. Gabapentin is a reference drug in the management of neuropathic pain, with at least 13 randomized controlled trials. Therefore, when used specifically for neuropathic pain, gabapentinoid AEDs may be considered primary analgesics and not simply adjuvants [28].

In a randomized, double-blind, active placebo-controlled crossover trial, patients with neuropathic pain received active placebo (lorazepam), sustained-release morphine, gabapentin, or a combination of gabapentin and morphine [30]. Each treatment was given orally for 5 weeks. The study indicated that the best analgesia was obtained from the gabapentin/morphine combination, with each medication given at a lower dose than that required when used as single agents.

Other studies have demonstrated that the concomitant administration of gabapentin reduces opioid requirements in the

Target	Medications	Actions
Serotonin and norepinephrine synaptic reuptake mechanisms in CNS	TCA, SSRI, SNRI	Enhance descending inhibition in CNS by blocking serotonin and norepinephrine reuptake
Na^+ channels (eg, tetrodotoxin-resistant sodium channel)	Lidocaine, mexiletine, lamotrigine, carbamazepine, phenytoin, doxepin, amitriptyline, other TCAs	Frequency-dependent blockade of depolarization; action on nociceptive DRG neurons
N-type Ca^{2+} channels ($\alpha_2\delta$ subunit)	Gabapentin, pregabalin	Suppress ectopic discharges in nociceptive DRG and dorsal horn neurons
GABA-B receptor	Baclofen	Agonist at the GABA-B receptors; enhances intraspinal inhibitory neurons
α_2 adrenoreceptors	Clonidine, tizanidine	Agonists at α_2 adrenoreceptors; inhibit neuropeptide release and ascending spinal pain transmission
NMDA receptors	D-methadone, dextromethorphan, memantine, ketamine	Antagonists at NMDA receptors; inhibit glutamate-mediated nociceptive transmission and prevent central sensitization
Osteoclasts	Bisphosphonates (eg, pamidronate, clodronate, zoledronic acid, ibandronate)	Apoptosis and inhibition of osteoclasts and other inflammatory and phagocytic cells
GR	Prednisone, methylprednisolone, dexamethasone	Agonists at peripheral intracellular GR; inhibit nociceptive immune mediators and inflammatory cell recruitment

Table 3. Common mechanisms of action for adjuvants. CNS: central nervous system; DRG: dorsal root ganglion; GABA: γ-aminobutyric acid; GR: glucocorticoid receptor; NMDA: N-methyl-D-aspartate; SNRI: serotonin and norepinephrine reuptake inhibitor; SSRI: selective serotonin reuptake inhibitor; TCA: tricyclic antidepressant; TRPV1: transient response potential vanilloid 1. *Continued overleaf.*

Target	Medications	Actions
Cannabinoid receptors	Dronabinol	Agonist at cannabinoid receptors; inhibits transmission at DRG
TRPV1 receptors	Capsaicin	Agonist at TRPV1; C-fiber neurotoxin; inactivates capsaicin-responsive nociceptors
Somatostatin	Octreotide	Agonist at somatostatin receptors; reduces vascular and nociceptive components of inflammation

Table 3. *Continued.*

postoperative setting [31,32]. Gabapentin has been found to be particularly effective in diabetic neuropathy, postherpetic neuralgia (PHN; for which it is approved by the FDA [33,34], and cancer neuropathies. Unfortunately, very few head-to-head studies against other AEDs or tricyclic antidepressants (TCAs) have been performed. Gabapentin has also been reported to be efficacious in neuropathic pain after spinal cord injury, Guillain–Barré syndrome, and postamputation phantom limb pain [35–37].

The side effects of gabapentin tend to occur early in treatment. The most common adverse events include dizziness, somnolence, and peripheral edema [29]. There is, however, considerable patient variation in tolerability, so gabapentin should be started at a low dosage and titrated gradually [38].

Case study: postinjury pain treated with gabapentin[a]
A 65-year-old man, working as a truck repairer, suffered severe maxillofacial trauma as a result of a crush injury at work. He incurred a fracture of the maxilla with significant displacement of the walls of the antrum and orbital floor. He subsequently underwent internal fixation with plates. He was referred to a pain clinic for multidisciplinary assessment. He described the

[a]Abridged with permission from the Pain Management Research Institute, 2005 (www.pmri.med.usyd.edu.au/ clinical/pdf/Resource_Orofacial4_Neuropathic.pdf).

pain as 'throbbing, shooting, stabbing, sharp, aching, splitting' on a pain questionnaire, and rated it 6 on a numeric rating scale (0 = no pain, 10 = worst pain imaginable). At the time of referral he was taking 2 g of acetaminophen daily. Carbamazepine had previously been tried, but was discontinued after 2 weeks due to excessive drowsiness. He reported a poor sleep pattern, with only 2 hours of sleep each night.

The patient was trialed on gabapentin, with an escalating dose up to 900 mg/day over 1 week. At his review appointment at 2 months he had achieved a 50% reduction in neuropathic facial pain by maintaining this regimen. He reported an occasional itch as the only side effect. He still complained of aching pain in the occipital region, which was attributed to coexisting C4/5 degenerative changes involving the facet joints.

Comment: The patient was a 'self-made' man, who had worked very hard over the years and built up his own business. The injury, hospitalization, and continuing pain had interfered with his business, and he sought 100% remission of facial and neck pain. Although his 50% response to gabapentin suggested an excellent early result, the patient remained disappointed and distress levels remained high.

The results of the early gabapentin trial gave rise to optimism that the pain problem could be impacted by appropriate medication over a period of time. At the same time, psychological rigidity of attitude and expectations, high stress, and unwillingness to adapt to less favorable physical conditions threatened to undermine the pharmacologic improvement.

Pregabalin

Pregabalin has been found to be effective in painful diabetic neuropathy, fibromyalgia, and PHN [39–41]. Pregabalin received FDA approval for the treatment of neuropathic pain in December 2004 and for the treatment of fibromyalgia in June 2007. It has a similar pharmacologic profile to gabapentin. However, pregabalin has a higher bioavailability than gabapentin (≥90% versus 27–60%) [29,42], and its plasma concentrations increase linearly as the dose is increased [42]. The side effects of pregabalin include weight gain, but otherwise are similar to those of gabapentin.

Nongabapentinoid antiepilepsy drugs
Carbamazepine and oxcarbazepine
Carbamazepine has an FDA indication for trigeminal neuralgia (a neuropathic condition characterized by brief, excruciating, lancinating pains). Carbamazepine is a Na^+ channel blocker. Adverse events such as dizziness, somnolence, unsteadiness, nausea and vomiting, and the need to monitor hematological function are significant drawbacks [43]. These have often influenced physicians to use newer and alternative AEDs (off-label) for trigeminal neuralgia, with a somewhat better toxicity profile than carbamazepine (eg, the keto-analog of carbamazepine, oxcarbazepine) [28].

Lamotrigine
A placebo-controlled trial found that lamotrigine was effective in controlling pain in refractory trigeminal neuralgia when combined with carbamazepine [44]. Lamotrigine has also shown some preliminary evidence of efficacy in neuropathies associated with human immune deficiency virus infection and poststroke pain. Unfortunately, in two recently conducted, replicate controlled studies, lamotrigine did not show consistent efficacy in the treatment of painful diabetic neuropathy [45]: in Study 2, the mean reduction in pain-intensity score from baseline to week 19 (the primary endpoint) was significantly greater in patients receiving lamotrigine 400 mg than in those receiving placebo; however, this was not replicated in Study 1. In addition, lamotrigine 300 and 400 mg were only occasionally more effective than placebo for secondary efficacy endpoints.

Dermatologic manifestations appear to be common with lamotrigine. In some cases, these are life-threatening. The risk of adverse effects can be reduced by titrating slowly from a small initial dose (25 mg/day) [2]. The benefit of lamotrigine might be due to the blockade of tetrodotoxin-resistant Na^+ channels.

Other antiepilepsy drugs

Valproic acid and topiramate have shown efficacy in the prevention and management of migraine headaches. Other AEDs (eg, zonisamide) might also have a role in the management of primary headaches [46].

Antidepressants

Antidepressants play an important role in the treatment of chronic pain. They display a wide variety of interactions with the neuraxis nociceptive pathways: monoamine modulation, descending inhibition, and ion-channel blocking [47].

McQuay et al. (1996) conducted a meta-analysis of 18 trials of antidepressants (all categories, total n=773) [48]. Compared with placebo, antidepressants provided:

- at least 50% pain relief in diabetic neuropathy
  (see **Figure 1**) – the best evidence was for desipramine
  and amitriptyline
- at least 50% pain relief in PHN
- at least 50% pain relief in atypical facial pain
- significantly greater benefit for all neuropathic conditions

Antidepressants with mixed reuptake transporter or norepinephrine activity appear to have the greatest analgesic effect in neuropathic pain. Predominantly serotonergic drugs, such as the selective serotonin reuptake inhibitors (SSRIs), are often ineffective in treating chronic pain.

Tricyclic antidepressants

For >30 years, antidepressants have been used off-label to manage neuropathic pain. There is, however, strong evidence that TCAs, in particular, are effective in the treatment of neuropathic pain syndromes such as PHN and diabetic neuropathy [49].

Sindrup and Jensen (2000) identified 10 placebo-controlled trials of TCAs (n=543) and calculated the number needed to

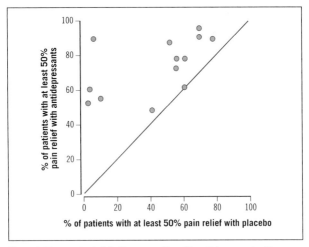

Figure 1. Treatment of diabetic neuropathy with antidepressants. The results are from a meta-analysis of 13 trials of antidepressants in diabetic neuropathy. For more details, see text.

Reproduced with permission from the International Association for the Study of Pain (McQuay JH, Tramèr M, Nye BA, et al. A systematic review of antidepressants in neuropathic pain. *Pain* 1996;68:217–27).

treat to obtain one patient with >50% pain relief [50]. They found that 2.6 patients must be treated with TCAs in order to obtain one patient with >50% pain relief, while 6.7 patients must be treated with SSRIs. They concluded that TCAs remain first line for the treatment of neuropathic pain.

TCAs (eg, amitriptyline, nortriptyline, desipramine) inhibit both serotonin and norepinephrine reuptake to varying degrees [28]. Of note, several TCAs (amitriptyline, doxepin, imipramine) have been found to have local anesthetic properties. Amitriptyline appears to be more potent than bupivacaine as a Na^+ channel blocker [51].

The use of TCAs should be closely monitored for frequent and often poorly tolerated adverse effects. These include sedation, dry mouth, constipation, and urinary retention [2]. Certain conditions may be aggravated by the use of TCAs, including heart disease, symptomatic prostatic hypertrophy, neurogenic bladder, dementia, and narrow-angle glaucoma. TCAs should be used with caution in patients with these conditions [2].

A baseline electrocardiogram is indicated for patients who are at risk of cardiac adverse effects, including elderly patients.

Serotonin and norepinephrine reuptake inhibitors

Serotonin and norepinephrine reuptake inhibitors (eg, duloxetine, venlafaxine) lack the anticholinergic and antihistamine effects of TCAs [28]. Duloxetine is FDA-approved for the treatment of pain secondary to diabetic neuropathy. Venlafaxine has also been shown to be effective in relieving pain associated with diabetic neuropathy [52]. Another antidepressant, bupropion, which inhibits the reuptake of dopamine, may be effective in the treatment of neuropathic pain [53].

Selective serotonin reuptake inhibitors

SSRIs (eg, paroxetine, fluoxetine) are effective antidepressants, but relatively ineffective analgesics [28]. While they are used for the management of comorbidities such as anxiety, depression, and insomnia, which frequently affect patients with chronic neuropathic pain, SSRIs have not shown the same efficacy as TCAs in the treatment of neuropathic pain [2].

Local anesthetics

Local anesthetics operate on the principle of decreasing neuronal excitability at the level of Na^+ channels that propagate action potentials. This channel blockade has an effect on both spontaneous and evoked pain. The analgesic properties occur at subanesthetic doses [28]. The FDA has approved transdermal lidocaine for the treatment of PHN.

Systemic local anesthetics can have a role in the treatment of central pain states [54]. The oral, antiarrhythmic, local anesthetic mexiletine has also been shown to have some analgesic properties in neuropathic pain. Mexiletine is contraindicated in the presence of second- and third-degree atrioventricular conduction blocks. Unfortunately, the incidence of GI side effects (eg, diarrhea, nausea) is quite high in patients taking mexiletine [54].

Of note, Na$^+$ channel-blocking properties are found not only in the traditional local anesthetics, but also in several AEDs (eg, carbamazepine, oxcarbazepine, lamotrigine) and TCAs (eg, amitriptyline, doxepin, imipramine) [55].

α_2-Adrenergic agonists

α_2-Adrenergic agonists are known to have a spinal antinociceptive effect. When given intrathecally, clonidine is known to potentiate the analgesic effect of opioids [28].

Tizanidine is a relatively short-acting, oral α_2-adrenergic agonist with a much lower hypotensive effect than clonidine. Tizanidine has been mostly used for the management of spasticity. However, some clinical observations indicate that tizanidine might have some usefulness in a variety of painful states, including neuropathic pain disorders [28].

Capsaicin

Capsaicin is the natural substance present in hot chili peppers. Capsaicin, along with heat and low pH, activates transient receptor potential vanilloid channels [56]. After an initial depolarization, a single administration of a large dose of capsaicin appears to produce a prolonged deactivation of a subgroup of pain fibers, also called capsaicin-sensitive nociceptors.

A systematic review of 16 studies has found capsaicin to be significantly more efficacious than placebo in the treatment of both musculoskeletal and neuropathic pain [57]. However, the efficacy was only poor to moderate. The authors concluded that capsaicin might be useful as an adjuvant or sole therapy in patients who are unresponsive to or intolerant of other treatments. The most common side effects of capsaicin are burning, stinging, and erythema at the application side, although these may diminish with use [57].

At the present time, preparations of injectable capsaicin and local anesthetics are being developed for site-specific, moderate to severe pain. These preparations should provide pain relief for patients with postsurgical, neuropathic, and musculoskeletal pain conditions for weeks or even months after a single treatment [28]. Preliminary clinical trials with injectable capsaicin and local anesthetics are currently underway for osteoarthritic pain and postsurgical pain following total knee replacement.

Case study: local treatment of postoperative pain[a]

A 55-year-old man underwent surgery for carcinoma of the soft palate. For the surgery, his mandible was split for access. Three months later, he complained of pain at the intraoral site of the incision passing over the mandibular alveolar crest. He described the pain as "very painful," indicating 6 on a numeric rating scale (0 = no pain, 10 = worst pain imaginable). He reported poor pain relief using a preparation containing 30 mg codeine and 300 mg acetaminophen per tablet, with an intake of 8 tablets daily.

The head and neck surgeon who carried out the operation initially thought that the pain was due to recurrence of the cancer, but there were no other features suggestive of recurrence. The surgeon referred the patient for pain relief. The patient received trials of amitriptyline 50 mg daily, carbamazepine 200 mg daily, and mexiletine 200 mg daily, but none was effective for pain relief and he discontinued them.

The patient underwent a trial of topical capsaicin that was applied to the site of the incision. For the trial he applied a topical anesthetic mouthrinse to the mucosa for 3 minutes, followed by a 3-minute application of 0.025% capsaicin cream. This was carried out morning and evening for 6 weeks. At his review appointment at 8 weeks he reported "very good pain relief" and he had completely ceased his codeine/ acetaminophen intake.

Comment: Although the medication selected by the patient's physician was appropriate, the dosages of all three drugs were

[a]Abridged with permission from the Pain Management Research Institute, 2005 (www.pmri.med.usyd.edu.au/clinical/pdf/Resource_Orofacial4_Neuropathic.pdf).

in the subtherapeutic range. It is likely that the patient would have gained benefit at dosages of mexiletine 200 mg three times daily, amitriptyline 75 mg at night, and carbamazepine 200 mg three times daily. The long-term use of codeine was not advisable, and the patient had continued to use it for 3 years despite only marginal benefit.

N-methyl-D-aspartate antagonists

Animal experiments show that central and peripheral *N*-methyl-D-aspartate (NMDA) receptors play an important role in hyperalgesia and chronic pain [58]. Glutamate is the dominant excitatory neurotransmitter in the mammalian CNS, and several lines of evidence indicate that central sensitization is mediated by NMDA receptors in the spinal cord [59].

Although studies of fixed-dose combinations of morphine/ dextromethorphan have failed to show enhanced opioid analgesia or decreased analgesic tolerance, the scientific interest in the study of NMDA antagonists in the management of hyperalgesic neuropathic states persists [60].

Dextromethorphan, D-methadone, memantine, amantadine, and ketamine all antagonize NMDA receptors. Ketamine, when used as an adjuvant to opioids, appears to increase pain relief by 20–30% and allows opioid dose reduction by 25–50% [61]. However, ketamine has a narrow therapeutic window and can cause intolerable side effects, such as hallucinations and memory impairment.

Of interest is the possibility that NMDA antagonists might prevent or counteract opioid analgesic tolerance [62].

Cannabinoids

The main therapeutic use of cannabinoids in humans is in the prevention of nausea and vomiting caused by chemotherapy. In patients with cancer or acquired immune deficiency syndrome, dronabinol or synthetic $\Delta(9)$-trans-tetrahydrocannabinol (Δ-9-THC) can be used to increase appetite and treat weight loss. Evidence from animal studies and clinical observations indicates that cannabinoids have some analgesic properties [63]. Δ-9-THC is the most widely studied cannabinoid. Analgesic sites of action have been identified in brain areas, in the spinal cord, and in the periphery. Cannabinoids appear to have a peripheral anti-inflammatory action, and to induce antinociception at lower doses than those obtained from effective CNS concentrations.

In contrast to the strong preclinical data, good clinical evidence on the efficacy of cannabinoids is still lacking. CNS depression seems to be the predominant limiting adverse effect. In chronic neuropathic pain, the cannabinoid compound CT-3, a THC-11-oic acid analog, has proven to be more effective than placebo [63].

Neuroimmunomodulatory agents

Several lines of evidence indicate that some proinflammatory ILs, such as tumor necrosis factor (TNF)-α, can play an important role in the genesis of inflammatory neuropathic pain [64]. Historically, glucocorticoids (eg, prednisone, methyl-prednisolone) have been employed to blunt the inflammatory response to tissue damage and, hence, pain. Aside from their disease-modifying actions (eg, limiting tissue damage in autoimmune disorders or altering tumor behavior/size), glucocorticoids provide analgesia through several mechanisms. The most important of these is switching off several inflammatory genes [65]. The net effect is a reduction in pronociceptive mediators, such as cytokines and PGs. The fact that initial (eg, posttraumatic) inflammatory phases can promote central sensitization has inspired several trials with glucocorticoids in the prevention of inflammatory neuropathic pain states. At this point, however, there is no clear consensus on their use.

The landscape of inflammatory and neuroimmune pain mediators is crowded. Nerve growth factor (NGF), TNF-α, IL-1β, IL-6, leukemia inhibitory factor, histamine, bradykinin, and PGE_2 can all produce pain when exogenously administered [64]. Of note, NGF has been shown to promote inflammatory neuropathic pain states. In the most recent animal models of cancer-related bone pain, anti-NGF therapy has been shown to produce a significant reduction in both ongoing and movement-related pain behavior. This treatment was more effective than morphine [66].

Neutralizing antibodies to TNF-α and IL-1 receptors could become an important therapeutic approach for severe inflammatory pain that is resistant to NSAIDs, as well as for forms of neuropathic pain [67].

Thalidomide has been shown to prevent hyperalgesia in animal models of neuropathic pain. Thalidomide is also known to inhibit TNF-α production. Newly developed TNF-α antagonists and thalidomide analogs with a better safety profile could play a role in the prevention and treatment of refractory inflammatory neuropathic painful disorders [68].

Finally, specific inhibitors of CNS microglia activation are being explored. These lines of research might open new and exciting treatment avenues [69].

γ-Aminobutyric acid agonists

Baclofen is an analog of the inhibitory neurotransmitter GABA. It has a specific action on the GABA-B receptors, and has been used for many years as a spasmolytic agent [70].

Clinical experience supports the use of low-dose baclofen to potentiate the antineuralgic effect of carbamazepine for trigeminal neuralgia. Baclofen has also been used intrathecally to relieve intractable spasticity, and it might have a role as an adjuvant when added to spinal opioids for the treatment of intractable neuropathic pain and spasticity [28].

The most common side effects of baclofen are drowsiness, weakness, hypotension, and confusion. Discontinuation of baclofen always requires a slow tapering in order to avoid seizures and other severe neurologic manifestations [28].

Bone metabolism modulators

Immunohistochemical studies have revealed an extensive network of nerve fibers in the vicinity of and within the skeleton. These are not only in the periosteum, but also in cortical and trabecular bone, as well as in the bone marrow [71]. Thinly myelinated and unmyelinated peptidergic sensory fibers, as well as sympathetic fibers, occur throughout the bone marrow, mineralized bone, and periosteum.

Bisphosphonates

There are numerous options for the treatment of bone pain. Bisphosphonate therapy has proven highly valuable in the management of numerous bone-related conditions, including hypercalcemia, osteoporosis, multiple myeloma, and Paget's disease. Bisphosphonates, synthetic analogs of pyrophosphate, bind with high affinity to bone hydroxyapatite crystals and reduce bone resorption by inhibiting osteoclastic activity [28].

Earlier bisphosphonates, such as etidronate, have been largely replaced by the use of second-generation (eg, pamidronate) and third-generation bisphosphonates (eg, zoledronic acid, ibandronate). Metastasis to bone is the most common cause of bone pain in cancer patients [72]. Bone pain is usually associated with direct tumor invasion of the bone, and is often severe and debilitating. Multiple studies have demonstrated the efficacy of second- and third-generation bisphosphonates in pain reduction for bone metastases [72].

Bisphosphonate treatment (eg, pamidronate, clodronate) has been reported to be efficacious not only in cancer-related bone pain, but also in the treatment of complex regional pain syndrome, a neuropathic inflammatory pain syndrome (see **Chapter 8**) [73]. Bisphosphonates suppress osteoclast-mediated bone resorption. The bisphosphonate analgesic effect is poorly understood. It might be related to the inhibition and apoptosis of activated phagocytic cells, such as osteoclasts and macrophages. This leads to a decreased release of proinflammatory cytokines in the area of inflammation.

One adverse event that has emerged in a number of cancer patients treated with the most potent bisphosphonates is osteonecrosis of the jaw. These patients were receiving bisphosphonate treatment for multiple myeloma or bone metastasis from breast, prostate, or lung cancer [74]. Risk factors for osteonecrosis of the jaw include prolonged duration of bisphosphonate treatment (ie, monthly IV administration for >1–2 years), poor oral hygiene, and a history of recent dental extraction [28].

Calcitonin

Calcitonin has several pain-related indications in patients who have bone pain, including osseous metastases. The most frequent routes of administration are intranasally and by subcutaneous injection. Calcitonin reduces bone resorption by inhibiting osteoclastic activity and osteolysis, and by an unknown central analgesic mechanism [28].

Adjuvants for visceral pain syndromes

The management of unrelenting visceral pain warrants the recognition of several unique features of visceral nociception:

- pain can be diffuse and poorly localized
- pain can be accompanied by motor and autonomic reflexes (eg, vomiting, diaphoresis, peristalsis)
- pain can manifest viscerosomatic convergence (referred pain)

In animal and human models, ketamine, an NMDA receptor antagonist, attenuates visceral pain [75]. Other adjuvants include somatostatin analogs and cannabinoids. Somatostatin appears to exhibit an anti-inflammatory and antinociceptive effect [76]. Octreotide, an octapeptide analog of somatostatin, has been used to treat carcinoid tumors. Octreotide has also been used off-label for visceral pain [77].

Summary

The management of severe neuropathic, bone, and visceral pain often represents a difficult treatment challenge. Although the pathophysiology of these conditions remains to be fully elucidated, treating multiple targets will probably be the standard of care.

The number and variety of adjuvants can be confusing, even for physicians who specialize in the treatment of pain. Physicians must know how to titrate the dose appropriately, while assessing the pain and managing drug-related side effects. Foremost, the treating physician needs to balance the efficacy, safety, and tolerability of several drugs, many of which will be employed off-label.

The physician who wishes to utilize adjuvants should keep abreast of the predominant mechanisms underlying difficult pain syndromes. As our knowledge of pain expands, so too will our arsenal of treatments.

References

1. World Health Organization. *Cancer Pain Relief*. Geneva: WHO, 1986.

2. Institute for Clinical Systems Improvement (ICSI). *Assessment and Management of Chronic Pain*. Bloomington: ICSI, 2005. Available from: www.icsi.org. Accessed August 30, 2007.

3. Shubhada NA, Kellie F, Subramanian P, et al., Editors. *The Washington Manual of Medical Therapeutics*, 31st edn. Philadelphia: Lippincott Williams & Wilkins, 2004.

4. van Tulder MW, Scholten RJ, Koes BW, et al. Non-steroidal anti-inflammatory drugs for low back pain. *Cochrane Database Syst Rev* 2000;(2):CD000396.

5. Vroomen P, de Krom M, Slofstra PD, et al. Conservative treatment of sciatica: a systematic review. *J Spinal Disord* 2000;13:463–9.

6. Elia N, Lysakowski C, Tramer MR. Does multimodal analgesia with acetaminophen, nonsteroidal antiinflammatory drugs, or selective cyclooxygenase-2 inhibitors and patient-controlled analgesia morphine offer advantages over morphine alone? Meta-analyses of randomized trials. *Anesthesiology* 2005;103:1296–304.

7. Marret E, Kurdi O, Zufferey P, et al. Effects of nonsteroidal antiinflammatory drugs on patient-controlled analgesia morphine side effects: meta-analysis of randomized trials. *Anesthesiology* 2005;102:1249–60.

8. Remy C, Marret E, Bonnet F. Effects of acetaminophen on morphine side-effects and consumption after major surgery: meta-analysis of randomized controlled trials. *Br J Anaesth* 2005;94:505–13.

9. McNicol E, Strassels SA, Goudas L, et al. NSAIDS or paracetamol, alone or combined with opioids, for cancer pain. *Cochrane Database Syst Rev* 2005;(1):CD005180.

10. Edwards JE, Oldman A, Smith L, et al. Single dose oral aspirin for acute pain. *Cochrane Database Syst Rev* 2000;(2):CD002067.

11. Sánchez-Delgado EJ. Life without COX2 inhibitors: risks and benefits are determined by dose and potency. *BMJ* 2006;17:1451–2.

12. Fored CM, Ejerblad E, Lindblad P, et al. Acetaminophen, aspirin, and chronic renal failure. *N Engl J Med* 2001;345:1801–8.

13. Brigden M, Smith RE. Acetylsalicylic-acid-containing drugs and nonsteroidal anti-inflammatory drugs available in Canada. *Can Med Assoc J* 1997;156:1025–8.

14. Jones R. Efficacy and safety of COX 2 inhibitors. *BMJ* 2002;325:607–8.

15. Laine L, Connors LG, Reicin A, et al. Serious lower gastrointestinal clinical events with nonselective NSAID or coxib use. *Gastroenterology* 2003;124:288–92.

16. Tannenbaum H, Bombardier C, Davis P, et al. For the Third Canadian Consensus Conference Group. An evidence-based approach to prescribing nonsteroidal antiinflammatory drugs. Third Canadian Consensus Conference. *J Rheumatol* 2006;33:140–57.

17. Moore RA, Derry S, Makinson GT, et al. Tolerability and adverse events in clinical trials of celecoxib in osteoarthritis and rheumatoid arthritis: systematic review and meta-analysis of information from company clinical trial reports. *Arthritis Res Ther* 2005;7:R644–65.

18. Silverstein FE, Faich G, Goldstein JL, et al. Gastrointestinal toxicity with celecoxib vs nonsteroidal anti-inflammatory drugs for osteoarthritis and rheumatoid arthritis: the CLASS study: a randomized controlled trial. Celecoxib Long-term Arthritis Safety Study. *JAMA* 2000;284:1247–55.

19. Bombardier C, Laine L, Reicin A, et al. For the VIGOR Study Group. Comparison of upper gastrointestinal toxicity of rofecoxib and naproxen in patients with rheumatoid arthritis. *N Engl J Med* 2000;343:1520–8.

20. Jüni P, Rutjes AW, Dieppe PA. Are selective COX 2 inhibitors superior to traditional non steroidal anti-inflammatory drugs? *BMJ* 2002;324:1287–8.

21. Topol EJ. Failing the public health – rofecoxib, Merck, and the FDA. *N Engl J Med* 2004;351:1707–9.

22. Kearney PM, Baigent C, Godwin J, et al. Do selective cyclo-oxygenase-2 inhibitors and traditional non-steroidal anti-inflammatory drugs increase the risk of atherothrombosis? Meta-analysis of randomised trials. *BMJ* 2006;332:1302–8.

23. Shaughnessy AF, Gordon AE. Life without COX 2 inhibitors. *BMJ* 2006;332:1287–8.

24. Bertolini A, Ferrari A, Ottani A, et al. Paracetamol: new vistas of an old drug. *CNS Drug Rev* 2006;12:250–75.

25. Bonnefont J, Daulhac L, Etienne M, et al. Acetaminophen recruits spinal p42/p44 MAPKs and GH/IGF-1 receptors to produce analgesia via the serotonergic system. *Mol Pharmacol* 2007;71:407–15.

26. McQuay H, Moore A, Justins D. Fortnightly review: Treating acute pain in hospital. *BMJ* 1997;314:1531–5

27. Watkins PB, Kaplowitz N, Slattery JT, et al. Aminotransferase elevations in healthy adults receiving 4 grams of acetaminophen daily: a randomized controlled trial. *JAMA* 2006;296:87–93.

28. Knotkova H, Pappagallo M. Adjuvant analgesics. *Med Clin N Am* 2007;91:113–24.

29. *Neurontin (Gabapentin): Prescribing Information.* Pfizer, Inc.

30. Gilron I, Bailey JM, Tu D, et al. Morphine, gabapentin, or their combination for neuropathic pain. *N Engl J Med* 2005;352:1324–34.

31. Eckhardt K, Ammon S, Hofmann U, et al. Gabapentin enhances the analgesic effect of morphine in healthy volunteers. *Anesth Analg* 2000;91:185–91.

32. Turan A, Karamanlioglu B, Memis D, et al. Analgesic effects of gabapentin after spinal surgery. *Anesthesiology* 2004;100:935–8.

33. Rowbotham M, Harden N, Stacey B, et al. Gabapentin for the treatment of postherpetic neuralgia: a randomized controlled trial. *JAMA* 1998;280:1837–42.

34. Rice AS, Maton S. Gabapentin in postherpetic neuralgia: a randomised, double blind, placebo controlled study. *Pain* 2001;94:215–24.

35. Bone M, Critchley P, Buggy DJ. Gabapentin in postamputation phantom limb pain: a randomized, double-blind, placebo-controlled, cross-over study. *Reg Anesth Pain Med* 2002;27:481–6.

36. Pandey CK, Bose N, Garg G, et al. Gabapentin for the treatment of pain in Guillain-Barré syndrome: a double-blinded, placebo-controlled, crossover study. *Anesth Analg* 2002;95:1719–23.

37. Tai Q, Kirshblum S, Chen B, et al. Gabapentin in the treatment of neuropathic pain after spinal cord injury: a prospective, randomized, double-blind, crossover trial. *J Spinal Cord Med* 2002;25:100–5.

38. Dworkin RH, Backonja M, Rowbotham MC, et al. Advances in neuropathic pain: diagnosis, mechanisms, and treatment recommendations. *Arch Neurol* 2003;60:1524–34.

39. Lesser H, Sharma U, LaMoreaux L, et al. Pregabalin relieves symptoms of painful diabetic neuropathy: a randomized controlled trial. *Neurology* 2004;63:2104–10.

40. Crofford LJ, Rowbotham MC, Mease PJ, et al. Pregabalin for the treatment of fibromyalgia syndrome: results of a randomized, double-blind, placebo-controlled trial. *Arthritis Rheum* 2005;52:1264–73.

41. Dworkin RH, Corbin AE, Young JP Jr, et al. Pregabalin for the treatment of postherpetic neuralgia: a randomized, placebo-controlled trial. *Neurology* 2003;60:1274–83.

42. *Lyrica (Pregabalin): Prescribing Information.* Pfizer, Inc.

43. *Tegretol (Carbamazepine): Prescribing Information.* Novartis, Inc.

44. Zakrzewska JM, Chaudhry Z, Nurmikko TJ, et al. Lamotrigine (Lamictal) in refractory trigeminal neuralgia: results from a double-blind placebo controlled crossover trial. *Pain* 1997;73:223–30.

45. Vinik AI, Tuchman M, Safirstein B, et al. Lamotrigine for treatment of pain associated with diabetic neuropathy: results of two randomized, double-blind, placebo-controlled studies. *Pain* 2007;128:169–79.

46. Pappagallo M. Newer antiepileptic drugs: possible uses in the treatment of neuropathic pain and migraine. *Clin Ther* 2003;25:2506–38.

47. Saarto T, Wiffen PJ. Antidepressants for neuropathic pain. *Cochrane Database Syst Rev* 2005;(3):CD005454.

48. McQuay HJ, Tramèr M, Nye BA, et al. A systematic review of antidepressants in neuropathic pain. *Pain* 1996;68:217–27.

49. McQuay HJ, Moore RA. Antidepressants and chronic pain. *BMJ* 1997;314:763–4.

50. Sindrup SH, Jensen TS. Pharmacologic treatment of pain in polyneuropathy. *Neurology* 2000;55:915–20.

51. Gerner P, Haderer AE, Mujtaba M, et al. Assessment of differential blockade by amitriptyline and its N-methyl derivative in different species by different routes. *Anesthesiology* 2003;98:1484–90.

52. Rowbotham MC, Goli V, Kunz NR, et al. Venlafaxine extended release in the treatment of painful diabetic neuropathy: a double-blind, placebo-controlled study. *Pain* 2004;110:697–706.

53. Semenchuk MR, Sherman S, Davis B. Double-blind, randomized trial of bupropion SR for the treatment of neuropathic pain. *Neurology* 2001;57:1583–8.

54. Tremont-Lukats IW, Challapalli V, McNicol ED, et al. Systemic administration of local anesthetics to relieve neuropathic pain: a systematic review and metaanalysis. *Anesth Analg* 2005;101:1738–49.

55. Lai J, Hunter JC, Porreca F. The role of voltage-gated sodium channels in neuropathic pain. *Curr Opin Neurobiol* 2003;13:291–7.

56. Caterina MJ, Schumacher MA, Tominaga M, et al. The capsaicin receptor: a heat-activated ion channel in the pain pathway. *Nature* 1997;389:816–24.

57. Mason L, Moore RA, Derry S, et al. Systematic review of topical capsaicin for the treatment of chronic pain. *BMJ* 2004;328:991–6.

58. Bennett AD, Everhart AW, Hulsebosch CE. Intrathecal administration of an NMDA or a non-NMDA receptor antagonist reduces mechanical but not thermal allodynia in a rodent model of chronic central pain after spinal cord injury. *Brain Res* 2000;859:72–82.

59. Dickenson AH, Chapman V, Green GM. The pharmacology of excitatory and inhibitory amino acid-mediated events in the transmission and modulation of pain in the spinal cord. *Gen Pharmacol* 1997;28:633–8.

60. Galer BS, Lee D, Ma T, et al. MorphiDex (morphine sulfate/dextromethorphan hydrobromide combination) in the treatment of chronic pain: three multicenter, randomized, double-blind, controlled clinical trials fail to demonstrate enhanced opioid analgesia or reduction in tolerance. *Pain* 2005;115:284–95.

61. Fitzgibbon EJ, Viola R. Parenteral ketamine as an analgesic adjuvant for severe pain: development and retrospective audit of a protocol for a palliative care unit. *J Palliat Med* 2005;8:49–57.

62. Price DD, Mayer DJ, Mao J, et al. NMDA-receptor antagonists and opioid receptor interactions as related to analgesia and tolerance. *J Pain Symptom Manage* 2000;19(Suppl. 1):S7–11.

63. Karst M, Salim K, Burstein S, et al. Analgesic effect of the synthetic cannabinoid CT-3 on chronic neuropathic pain: a randomized controlled trial. *JAMA* 2003;290:1757–62.

64. Marchand F, Perretti M, McMahon SB. Role of the immune system in chronic pain. *Nat Rev Neurosci* 2005;6:521–32.

65. Barnes PJ. Anti-inflammatory actions of glucocorticoids: molecular mechanisms. *Clin Sci (London)* 1998;94:557–72.

66. Sevcik MA, Ghilardi JR, Peters CM, et al. Anti-NGF therapy profoundly reduces bone cancer pain and the accompanying increase in markers of peripheral and central sensitization. *Pain* 2005;115:128–41.

67. Schafers M, Brinkhoff J, Neukirchen S, et al. Combined epineurial therapy with neutralizing antibodies to tumor necrosis factor-alpha and interleukin-1 receptor has an additive effect in reducing neuropathic pain in mice. *Neurosci Lett* 2001;310:113–16.

68. Goli V. Does thalidomide have an analgesic effect? Current status and future directions. *Curr Pain Headache Rep* 2007;11:109–14.

69. D'Acquisto F, May MJ, Ghosh S. Inhibition of nuclear factor kappa B (NF-kappaB): an emerging theme in anti-inflammatory therapies. *Mol Interv* 2002;2:22–35.

70. Chou R, Peterson K, Helfand M. Comparative efficacy and safety of skeletal muscle relaxants for spasticity and musculoskeletal conditions: a systematic review. *J Pain Symptom Manage* 2004;28:140–75.

71. Lerner UH. Neuropeptidergic regulation of bone resorption and bone formation. *J Musculoskelet Neuronal Interact* 2002;2:440–7.

72. Slatkin N. Cancer-related pain and its pharmacologic management in the patient with bone metastasis. *J Support Oncol* 2006;4(Suppl.):15–21.

73. Pappagallo M. Bisphosphonate therapy for non-cancer pain. *Adv Pain Manage* 2007;1:19–23.

74. Bamias A, Kastritis E, Bamia C, et al. Osteonecrosis of the jaw in cancer after treatment with bisphosphonates: incidence and risk factors. *J Clin Oncol* 2005;23:8580–7.

75. Strigo IA, Duncan GH, Bushnell MC, et al. The effects of racemic ketamine on painful stimulation of skin and viscera in human subjects. *Pain* 2005;113:255–64.

76. Helyes Z, Than M, Oroszi G, et al. Anti-nociceptive effect induced by somatostatin released from sensory nerve terminals and by synthetic somatostatin analogues in the rat. *Neurosci Lett* 2000;278:185–8.

77. Hornby PJ, Prouty SM. Involvement of cannabinoid receptors in gut motility and visceral perception. *Br J Pharmacol* 2004;141:1335–45.

14 • Opioids

For centuries, opioids have been used as effective remedies in the management of moderate to severe pain. Interestingly, targeted pharmaceutical research in analgesic therapy over the last 50 years has not been particularly successful, either in increasing analgesic efficacy or in decreasing the incidence of adverse effects. The clinical management of moderate to severe chronic pain still depends on old drugs or combinations of derivatives of old drugs, such as morphine and aspirin. Exceptions are the anticonvulsants (eg, gabapentin, pregabalin) and antidepressants (eg, duloxetine), which seem to have improved the control of neuropathic pain.

Examples of the more commonly used opioids are tramadol, hydrocodone, morphine, oxycodone, oxymorphone, fentanyl, hydromorphone, buprenorphine, and methadone.

When is it appropriate to use opioids?

There have been increasing concerns about the serious adverse effects of both selective and nonselective nonsteroidal anti-inflammatory drugs (NSAIDs) (see **Chapter 13**). For example, a recent meta-analysis concluded that both cyclooxygenase inhibitors and the nonselective NSAIDs (except for naproxen) are associated with a 40% increased risk of serious vascular events compared with placebo [1].

Acetaminophen is an obvious alternative to NSAIDs, but dose titration is limited by hepatotoxicity, and it cannot provide sufficient pain relief in the management of disabling inflammatory conditions, including osteoarthritis and rheumatoid arthritis. This has left physicians with fewer options in the treatment of many patients with chronic painful conditions.

The careful use of opioid analgesics should be considered in the treatment of pain when nonopioid analgesics (acetaminophen and low-dose NSAIDs) and nonpharmacologic options have proven inadequate for pain control [2]. When medically appropriate, opioid analgesics can be recommended for chronic, moderate to severe disabling pain [2]. This can be defined, for practical purposes, as a pain score >4 on the Brief Pain Inventory pain intensity scale of 0–10 (see **Chapter 3**).

Opioids are still considered as the most potent and effective 'broad-spectrum' analgesics in the treatment of chronic pain. As such, they have been prescribed to patients suffering from moderate to severe disabling pain of both cancer and noncancer origin.

Morphine, a μ-agonist that was isolated from opium >100 years ago, represents the mainstay for the treatment of moderate to severe cancer pain. The analgesic action of other opioid agonists is well known and utilized clinically in pain management.

The efficacy of opioids in chronic noncancer pain, including pain and associated disability related to a variety of neuropathic pain syndromes, has been established in a number of randomized controlled trials [3–17].

Pharmacology and clinical use

Opioids are agonists that act on opioid receptors in the peripheral and central nervous systems (CNS). Endogenous ligands include β-endorphins, met-enkephalins, and dynorphins. A number of receptors that are responsible for opioid effects have been characterized. These include μ-, δ-, and κ-receptors.

Morphine has a very high affinity for the μ-receptor, while oxycodone has an additional affinity for the κ-receptor, a receptor that has been implicated in the attenuation of hypersensitivity in certain visceral pain states in experimental pain models [18]. Buprenorphine is a partial μ-agonist and a κ-antagonist.

The opioids have peripheral, spinal, and supraspinal targets. At the presynaptic neuronal level, opioids reduce Ca^{2+} influx in the primary nociceptive afferents, resulting in decreased neurotransmitter release. At the postsynaptic level, opioids enhance K^+ efflux, resulting in hyperpolarization of the dorsal horn pain-signaling sensory neurons. The net result of the opioid action is a decrease in nociceptive transmission.

It is now recognized that opioids can exert analgesic effects at peripheral sites. Of note, the opioid peripheral effect on primary nociceptive afferents might play a relevant role during painful inflammatory states [19,20]. In the midbrain, opioids will activate so-called 'off' cells and inhibit 'on' cells, leading to activation of a descending inhibitory control on spinal neurons [21].

The goal of opioid therapy is to provide analgesia and to maintain or improve function, with minimal side effects. The indications for the use of opioids in moderate to severe chronic pain of nonmalignant origin are osteoarthritis, musculoskeletal pain, and neuropathic pain, with the common denominator that various pharmacologic and nonpharmacologic procedures have proved unsuccessful [22,23].

Which opioid should be used?

It is crucial to recognize that the potency and effectiveness of different opioids will differ between patients. Variability among patients can be quite profound. This can extend towards both the analgesic effects and the side effects [24]. Predicting a patient's response to medication has long been a goal of clinicians; it is probable that the new science of pharmacogenomics will, in due course, allow screening for variations in the expression of drug-metabolizing enzymes (eg, cytochrome [CY]P2D6, CYP3A4), and thus provide a potent tool for improving pain management.

> All physicians who are prescribing opioids should be acquainted with at least two different opioids.

Sustained-release (SR) opioid preparations currently available are: oral tramadol, oral morphine, oral oxycodone, oral oxymorphone, and transdermal fentanyl. Immediate-release (IR) or fast-acting preparations currently available are: tramadol, oral hydrocodone (available only in combination with acetaminophen or NSAIDs), transmucosal fentanyl (available as oral transmucosal fentanyl citrate or a fentanyl buccal tablet), oral oxymorphone, oral oxycodone, oral morphine, and oral hydromorphone. Both methadone and buprenorphine have long-acting analgesic properties.

Opioid therapy for patients with chronic noncancer pain should rely on SR preparations associated with a well-defined daily number of IR opioid rescue doses for breakthrough pain (note: this is contrary to the treatment recommendations in cancer pain, where fairly unrestricted access to rescue doses is advisable). Outside the palliative care and cancer pain outpatient practices, long-term use of intramuscular or intravenous opioid injections for ambulatory and otherwise relatively functional patients with chronic pain should be discouraged.

Tramadol

Tramadol has weak μ-agonist properties [25,26]. Tramadol inhibits reuptake of the monoamines norepinephrine and serotonin [25,26], an analgesic mechanism comparable with that of tricyclic antidepressants, serotonin and norepinephrine reuptake inhibitors, and selective serotonin reuptake inhibitors. Analgesic efficacy has been demonstrated in neuropathic pain [26].

Tramadol is not a controlled substance. It is available in both IR (50 mg) and SR (100, 200, or 300 mg) oral preparations. The bioavailability is 75% and 85–90%, respectively [27,28]. Tramadol is also available in a tablet in combination with acetaminophen (37.5 mg tramadol and 325 mg acetaminophen).

Morphine

The World Health Organization has placed morphine on the Essential Drug List. Morphine is the opioid of reference, particularly in cancer pain, but a number of important alternatives exist [29]. Morphine can be administered topically, orally, or parenterally (including by the spinal route). There are four oral formulations: elixir, IR tablets, SR tablets, or capsules (15–200 mg). Following oral ingestion, the systemic bioavailability is <40% due to extensive presystemic elimination in the liver [30]. With most opioids, including morphine, the effect of a given dose is less after oral than after parenteral administration because of variable but significant first-pass metabolism in the liver. For example, the bioavailability of oral preparations of morphine is only about 25%. The shape of the time–effect curve also varies with the route of administration, so the duration of action often is somewhat longer with the oral route. If adjustment is made for variability of first-pass metabolism and clearance, adequate relief of pain can be achieved with oral administration of morphine. Satisfactory analgesia in cancer patients is associated with a very broad range of steady-state concentrations of morphine in plasma (16–364 ng/mL) [31]. When morphine and most opioids are given intravenously, they act promptly. However, the more lipid-soluble compounds act more rapidly than morphine after subcutaneous administration because of differences in the rates of absorption and entry into the CNS.

Morphine is metabolized to two major metabolites: morphine-3-glucuronide (M3G) and an active analgesic metabolite, morphine-6-glucuronide (M6G) [30]. M6G has a longer elimination half-life than morphine (2 hours), and the duration of analgesia for IR preparations is therefore 3–4 hours.

Elimination depends primarily on kidney function, but impaired hepatic function can also lead to the accumulation of morphine or morphine metabolites [30]. M3G has a low affinity for opioid receptors and may contribute to the excitatory effects of morphine. Some investigators have shown that M3G can antagonize morphine-induced analgesia [32]. M3G can accumulate in renal insufficiency, leading to myoclonus and fasciculations, and is thought to contribute to the development of hyperalgesia.

Hydrocodone

Hydrocodone is a µ-agonist that is thought to be equipotent to morphine for pain control in humans. Hydrocodone is not available as a single agent; reportedly, there are >200 products containing hydrocodone (usual doses in tablets are 5, 7.5, and 10 mg). In its most common preparations, hydrocodone is not only combined with acetaminophen, but also with aspirin, ibuprofen, and antihistamines. It is available as an elixir formulation.

Oxycodone

Oxycodone, a synthetic opioid, has been in use as an analgesic since the early 1920s [33]. Lower doses of oxycodone, in combination with acetaminophen or aspirin, have been extensively used for the treatment of pain of mild to moderate intensity. Oxycodone is in part metabolized through CYP450 2D6 [34]. Approximately 5–10% of the white population is deficient in 2D6 activity, and many medications, including antidepressants and antiepilepsy drugs, are metabolized through CYP2D6. Thus, drug–drug interactions and deficiency in CYP2D6 activity might affect pain relief in some patients [34].

Oxycodone has a bioavailability of >60% [34]. The median equianalgesic ratio between oral morphine and oxycodone is 2:1. Oxycodone is available as an elixir, IR capsules, and SR tablets (5–80 mg). The SR formulation contains IR oxycodone on the surface of the tablet, which might give a faster onset of action than traditional SR formulations.

Three placebo-controlled trials have demonstrated analgesic efficacy for oxycodone in diabetic neuropathy and postherpetic neuralgia [11,12,35].

Oxymorphone

Oxymorphone is a semisynthetic μ-opioid agonist. The Food and Drug Administration first approved oxymorphone in 1959 [36]. IR (5 or 10 mg) and SR (5, 10, 20, or 40 mg) oral formulations of this drug are available. Oxymorphone SR is three times as potent as morphine, but has poor oral bioavailability (10%). Whereas oxycodone may have activity at more than one receptor subtype (ie, μ- and κ-receptors), oxymorphone exhibits insignificant interaction with κ- or δ-receptors, but binds with high affinity to μ-receptors [37]. In terms of equianalgesia and opioid conversion, the oral oxycodone:oxymorphone ratio is 2:1, and the oral morphine:oxymorphone ratio is 3:1 [38].

Hydromorphone

Oral hydromorphone is four times as potent as morphine. Hydromorphone has traditionally been used in the palliative care setting in patients who require high doses of opioids; however, it has increasingly become an alternative to other opioids in the management of severe postoperative pain and cancer pain. Hydromorphone is approximately 50% bioavailable when given orally and is available in tablets (2, 4, and 8 mg), in oral solution (5 mg/5 mL), and as a rectal suppository (3 mg).

Fentanyl

Fentanyl belongs to a group of opioids in use in anesthesia and intensive care, due to their rapid onset and short duration of action. Fentanyl has high lipid solubility, low molecular weight, and high potency, making it suitable for a transdermal preparation. Fentanyl is available as a long-acting transdermal patch (12–100 μg/hour), as IR, fast-acting, transmucosal buccal tablets (100–800 μg; 65% bioavailability), or as a medicated lozenge on a stick (200–1,600 μg; 50% bioavailability).

For the fentanyl patch, the time from initial application to a stable plasma concentration is 12–24 hours due to the slow build-up of a subcutaneous reservoir. Peak plasma concentrations are obtained between 24 and 72 hours after the initial application; following removal of the patch, a residual depot is present so that, on average, plasma concentrations fall by 50% in 17 hours [39].

Buprenorphine

Buprenorphine is an interesting synthetic opioid that was originally introduced into clinical practice as a parenteral analgesic in anesthesia. Buprenorphine is a partial μ-opioid high-affinity receptor agonist and a κ-opioid receptor antagonist. The bioavailability following oral administration is very low. Like fentanyl, buprenorphine has high lipid solubility, low molecular weight, and high potency. It is available sublingually. Since the 1980s, buprenorphine has been associated with an analgesic 'ceiling effect', bringing into question its analgesic efficacy in severe and rapidly progressing pain.

Under the Drug Addiction Treatment Act of 2000, buprenorphine HCL and buprenorphine HCL plus naloxone sublingual tablets (2 or 8 mg buprenorphine, with or without 0.5 or 2 mg naloxone, respectively) can be prescribed by qualified physicians for the office-based treatment of opiate dependence (opioid addiction). Both a summary and the full text of the Act are available from the Department of Health & Human Services at www.hhs.gov.

Methadone

Methadone is the most inexpensive oral opioid agent available. It is a racemic mixture of d- and l-methadone. It has antagonistic activity at the noncompetitive N-methyl-D-aspartate receptor site [40]. Methadone is available as a tablet (5 and 10 mg) and diskette (40 mg tablet). Oral methadone has excellent, although highly variable, bioavailability (50–100%). Its pharmacokinetic profile is affected by plasma protein (α_1-glycoprotein) binding and CYP3A4 activity [41]. CYP3A4 inhibitors (eg, diazepam, fluoxetine, paroxetine, verapamil) can increase methadone serum levels, while CYP3A4 inducers (eg, dexamethasone, carbamazepine, phenytoin, isoniazid, topiramate) can decrease its levels.

The potency of methadone increases as the total daily dose of morphine increases; therefore, a variable conversion ratio exists from morphine to methadone. This varies according to the daily morphine dose (see **Table 1**) [40].

There is an association between methadone and QT prolongation and torsades de pointes. This may be more frequent with intravenous methadone or with high oral doses of methadone (>200 mg/day), concomitant administration of CYP3A4 inhibitors, hypokalemia, hepatic failure, administration of other QT-prolonging drugs and pre-existing heart disease [42,43].

Methadone has a long and variable half-life, which predisposes to drug accumulation [40]; methadone should therefore be used cautiously and only by clinicians who are experienced with its use.

Opioid-related adverse effects

The assessment and management of adverse effects is an essential part of opioid therapy. By adequately treating adverse effects, it is often possible to titrate the opioid to a higher dose and thereby increase the responsiveness of the pain [44]. Because different opioids can produce different adverse effects in a given patient, opioid rotation (see the next section) is an option for the treatment of persistent adverse effects.

Opioid bowel dysfunction

Opioid bowel dysfunction (OBD) is a common adverse effect associated with opioid therapy. OBD is commonly described as constipation; however, it refers to a constellation of adverse gastrointestinal (GI) effects, which also includes abdominal cramping, bloating, gastroesophageal reflux, and gastroparesis. The mechanism for these effects is mediated primarily by stimulation of opioid receptors in the GI tract. In patients with pain, uncontrolled symptoms of OBD can add to their discomfort and may serve as a barrier to effective pain management by limiting therapy or prompting discontinuation [45]. Prophylactic treatment should be provided for constipation. Constipation can be managed with a stepwise approach that includes an increase in fiber and fluids and osmotic agents (eg, sorbitol, lactulose), or with a combination stool softener and a mild peristaltic stimulant laxative such as senna or bisacodyl, as needed [2].

Promising studies are investigating the efficacy of peripherally acting opioid antagonist compounds (eg, alvimopan, methylnaltrexone) [46]. These agents, while effectively treating OBD, do not inhibit the central analgesic effects of opioids. Alvimopan has a very low systemic absorption and specifically antagonizes the μ-opioid receptors in the GI tract. Methylnaltrexone is a derivative of naltrexone. It does not cross the blood–brain barrier and therefore acts only as a selective peripheral opioid antagonist, blocking the μ-receptors in the GI tract. Oral naloxone, which has minimal systemic absorption, has also been used empirically to treat constipation without reversing analgesia in most cases [47].

Nausea and vomiting

A meta-analysis of opioids in moderate to severe noncancer pain found nausea to affect 21% of patients [48]. Opioids can cause dizziness, nausea, and vomiting by stimulating the medullary chemoreceptor trigger zone, increasing the inner ear vestibular system (ie, motion sickness), or inducing gastroparesis (or even retroperistalsis, both part of OBD) [49]. With vomiting, parenteral administration of antiemetics may be required. If nausea is caused by gastric stasis, treatment is similar to that of OBD. Tolerance to nausea usually develops.

Drowsiness

Daytime drowsiness is frequent at the initiation of opioid therapy, but can be minimized by using a low starting dose and titrating progressively. If somnolence does occur, it usually subsides within a few days as tolerance develops. The use of a psychostimulant (eg, methylphenidate, dextroamphetamine) can be considered if persistent somnolence has a detrimental effect on the patient's functioning [49].

Delirium

Delirium is frequent in elderly patients, particularly those with cognitive impairment [49]. It can be prevented or treated by using low doses of IR opioids and discontinuing other CNS-acting drugs.

Hypogonadism

Hypogonadism (low testosterone serum levels) can occur in male patients [2]. The testosterone level should be verified in patients who complain of sexual dysfunction or other symptoms of hypogonadism (eg, fatigue, anxiety, depression). Testosterone supplementation is effective in treating hypogonadism, but close monitoring of the testosterone serum level as well as screening for benign prostate hypertrophy and prostate cancer should be carried out.

Respiratory depression

Although respiratory depression fosters the greatest concern, tolerance to this adverse effect develops rapidly. Respiratory depression is very uncommon if the opioid is titrated according to accepted dosing guidelines [50].

What is opioid rotation? When and how should it be done?

Opioid rotation refers to the switch from one opioid to another, and it is recommended when adverse effects or onset of analgesic tolerance limit the degree of analgesia obtained

Drug	Route	Ratio (oral morphine:opioid)	Example
Morphine	PO	1:1	
Hydromorphone	PO	4:1	30 mg morphine = 7.5 mg hydromorphone
Oxycodone	PO	2:1	30 mg morphine = 15 mg oxycodone
Oxymorphone	PO	3:1	30 mg morphine = 10 mg oxymorphone
Tramadol	PO	1:6	30 mg morphine = 200 mg tramadol
Hydrocodone	PO	1:1	30 mg morphine = 30 mg hydrocodone
Methadone	PO	4:1 (with morphine daily dose 30–90 mg)	30 mg morphine = 7.5 mg methadone
		8:1 (with morphine daily dose 91–300 mg)	300 mg morphine = 35 mg methadone
		12:1 (with morphine daily dose >300 mg)	400 mg morphine = 35 mg methadone

Table 1. Opioid conversion table. PO: by mouth.
Adapted from Manfredi PL, Houde RW. Prescribing methadone, a unique analgesic. *J Support Oncol* 2003;1:216–20.

with the current opioid [2]. This approach is based on the observation that a patient's response varies from opioid to opioid, both for analgesia and adverse effects. Therefore, the absence of an analgesic response or the occurrence of an adverse effect with one opioid does not predict a similar response to another opioid. According to clinical experience, observations, and case reports, opioid rotation results in clinical improvement in >50% of patients with chronic pain who have had a poor response to one opioid [51].

Opioid rotation should always be based on an equianalgesic opioid conversion table, which provides evidence-based values for the relative potencies among different opioid drugs. **Table 1** shows dose equivalents for some commonly used opioids [52]. The first step is to determine the patient's current total daily opioid utilization. This can be accomplished by adding up the doses of all long-acting and short-acting opioids consumed by the patient per day. If the patient is on multiple opioids, convert all of them to morphine equivalents using standard equianalgesic tables. Usually, when switching from opioid A to opioid B, it is prudent to decrease the equianalgesic dose of opioid B by 50–67%. If opioid B is methadone, the dose should be reduced by a greater amount, eg, by approximately 93%, given in divided doses every 8 hours, if switching from morphine 200–500 mg/day [2].

The dose of opioid B should also be adjusted based on clinical circumstances. For example, the dose of opioid B might be reduced even further in patients who are elderly or who have significant cardiopulmonary, hepatic, or renal disease. In contrast, if the patient complains of severe pain, the dose may be administered at the equianalgesic dose, without any dose reduction. The patient must remain under close clinical supervision to prevent overdose.

Under supervision, a safe, effective, and rapid opioid rotation and titration can be performed via intravenous patient-controlled analgesia. This option should be considered for patients with severe disabling pain who are on large daily doses of opioids, including oral methadone or multiple opioids, and for frail or elderly patients.

Are opioids effective in neuropathic pain?

Opioid responsiveness is defined as the achievement of adequate analgesia with an opioid dose that is not associated with intolerable side effects. The responsiveness of neuropathic pain to opioids has long been an area of controversy, with some considering it as inherently resistant.

Based on current scientific knowledge and clinical experience, a consensus has now been reached: although neuropathic pain might be less responsive to opioids than nociceptive pain, some degree of analgesia can be reached with a well-tolerated dose [53,54].

Evidence from multiple randomized controlled trials indicates that opioids (SR morphine, SR oxycodone, methadone, levorphanol, and tramadol) can relieve pain and associated disability in a variety of neuropathic pain syndromes [2]. Opioid analgesics have an established role in the contemporary treatment algorithm for neuropathic pain, and should therefore be used in the management of the patient with disabling, moderate to severe, neuropathic pain [55].

> Although neuropathic pain may be less responsive to opioids than nociceptive pain, some degree of analgesia can be reached with a well-tolerated dose.

Opioids in older patients

Due to frequent comorbidities and polypharmacy, as well as increased frailty, older patients are more prone to adverse effects from opioids [22]. Concerns regarding adverse effects are held by healthcare professionals, patients, and patients' families, and can prevent older patients from receiving adequate pain control. Unfortunately, untreated pain also has a detrimental effect on older people, including reduced physical functioning, depression, sleep impairment, and decreased quality of life. The inadequate management of postoperative pain has also been shown to be a risk factor for delirium.

Most opioid analgesics can be used safely and effectively in older patients, providing the regimen is adapted to each patient's specificities and comorbidities (eg, the presence of renal or hepatic failure, dementia). As in all patients, regardless of age, the opioid should be started at the lowest available dose and titrated slowly, depending on analgesic response and adverse effects [2].

SR, long-acting formulations can be used safely, but they should only be given to patients for whom an effective and safe daily dose of a short-acting opioid has been established. The efficacy of the opioid should be re-evaluated on a regular basis and it should be discontinued if not effective. The presence of adverse effects should be assessed systematically, and they should be treated where possible. For frequent adverse effects, it might be appropriate to institute a preventive regimen (eg, a prophylactic bowel regimen in patients at risk of constipation).

Some opioids, such as meperidine and propoxyphene, should not be used in older patients [22]. The active metabolite of meperidine (normeperidine) accumulates, and is associated with a high occurrence of psychomimetic effects, as well as rare occurrences of seizures. Propoxyphene has similar properties and therefore carries the same concerns, although to a lesser degree.

Nonopioid analgesics (eg, acetaminophen), adjuvant analgesics, and nonpharmacologic treatments (eg, physical therapy, exercise) should be used concurrently with opioid therapy [22]. These will reduce the opioid dose that is required to achieve analgesia, and hence reduce the associated adverse effects.

Opioid therapy: patient education

Patient education is an essential part of opioid therapy; it should begin before therapy is instituted, and continue throughout the course of treatment. Components of an educational information sheet for the patient usually include the following points [56]:

- Opioids are powerful pain-relieving drugs, and are effective in a number of painful disorders. However, they are strictly regulated and must be used as directed, and only by the person for whom they are prescribed.

- The goals of pain management are to help you (the patient) feel better and live a more active life. This usually takes more than medication: nondrug treatments such as physical therapy, relaxation, and exercise can also be of use.
- If you stop these medicines suddenly then your body might react physically. When stopping these medicines, you should taper them off gradually and only on your physician's advice.
- Common side effects include nausea, dry mouth, drowsiness with cognitive impairment, impaired voiding, and itchy skin. These usually last 1–2 weeks until tolerance develops. They can be managed. Nausea and itch may be prevented by antiemetics (eg, ondansetron, diphenhydramine). Constipation does not go away, but can usually be managed by eating the right foods, drinking enough liquids, and, as a rule, always taking laxatives. Osmotic laxatives such as lactulose, stool softeners such as polyethylene glycol, or peristalsis stimulators such as sodium picosulfate prescribed twice daily are effective.
- Work with your pain management team. Ask what you can do to take a more active part in your healthcare.

A patient information sheet can be downloaded from www.ohsu.edu/ahec/pain/patientinformation.pdf.

Opioid therapeutic trial

It is recommended that the patient undergo one or more therapeutic trials of opioids prior to making a decision regarding long-term therapy. This could be in the form of a 12-week trial period of the planned therapy with oral opioids. During the trial, the patient should undergo frequent reviews to achieve dose titration and to assess clinical efficacy.

Opioid doses should be titrated up until the patient experiences adequate pain relief. Adequate analgesia must be balanced against side effects. There is no ceiling dose for most opioids; doses should be increased according to clinical need, and under regular and careful monitoring for analgesic efficacy and adverse effects.

If the patient does not receive adequate pain relief from one opioid, or if the patient experiences intolerable side effects, it may be necessary to switch the patient to an alternative opioid (opioid rotation).

Risk management is extremely important with opioids. Essential risk management strategies are detailed in **Chapter 15**.

> Opioid rotation should be considered either when inadequate analgesia is obtained or when intolerable side effects appear.

Summary

Opioids should be considered very valuable analgesics. They should be used in combination with other pharmacologic and nonpharmacologic methods in the management of chronic pain of nonmalignant origin.

References

1. Kearney PM, Baigent C, Godwin J, et al. Do selective cyclo-oxygenase-2 inhibitors and traditional non-steroidal anti-inflammatory drugs increase the risk of atherothrombosis? Meta-analysis of randomised trials. *BMJ* 2006;332:1302–8.

2. Veterans Health Administration, Department of Defense. *VA/DoD Clinical Practice Guideline for the Management of Opioid Therapy for Chronic Pain.* Washington: Veterans Health Administration, Department of Defense, 2003.

3. Arkinstall W, Sandler A, Goughnour B, et al. Efficacy of controlled-release codeine in chronic non-malignant pain: a randomized, placebo-controlled clinical trial. *Pain* 1995;62:169–78.

4. Peloso PM, Bellamy N, Bensen W. Double blind randomized placebo controlled trial of controlled release codeine in the treatment of osteoarthritis of the hip and knee. *J Rheumatol* 2000;27:764–71.

5. Roth SH, Fleischmann RM, Burch FX, et al. Around-the-clock, controlled-release oxycodone therapy for osteoarthritis-related pain: placebo-controlled trial and long-term evaluation. *Arch Intern Med* 2000;160:853–60.

6. Caldwell JR, Hale ME, Boyd RE, et al. Treatment of osteoarthritis pain with controlled release oxycodone or fixed combination oxycodone plus acetaminophen added to nonsteroidal antiinflammatory drugs: a double blind, randomized, multicenter, placebo controlled trial. *J Rheumatol* 1999;26:862–9.

7. Caldwell JR, Rapoport RJ, Davis JC, et al. Efficacy and safety of a once-daily morphine formulation in chronic, moderate-to-severe osteoarthritis pain: results from a randomized, placebo-controlled, double-blind trial and an open-label extension trial. *J Pain Symptom Manage* 2002;23:278–91.

8. Allan L, Hays H, Jensen NH, et al. Randomised crossover trial of transdermal fentanyl and sustained release oral morphine for treating chronic non-cancer pain. *BMJ* 2001;322:1154–8.

9. Jamison RN, Raymond SA, Slawsby EA, et al. Opioid therapy for chronic noncancer back pain. A randomized prospective study. *Spine* 1998;23:2591–600.

10. Moulin DE, Iezzi A, Amireh R, et al. Randomised trial of oral morphine for chronic non-cancer pain. *Lancet* 1996;347:143–47.

11. Gimbel JS, Richards P, Portenoy RK. Controlled-release oxycodone for pain in diabetic neuropathy: a randomized controlled trial. *Neurology* 2003;60:927–34.

12. Watson CP, Babul N. Efficacy of oxycodone in neuropathic pain: a randomized trial in postherpetic neuralgia. *Neurology* 1998;50:1837–41.

13. Dellemijn P, Vanneste J. Randomized double-blind active-placebo-controlled crossover trial of intravenous fentanyl in neuropathic pain. *Lancet* 1997;349:753–8.

14. Raja S, Haythornthwaite J, Pappagallo M, et al. Opioids versus antidepressants in postherpetic neuralgia: a randomized-placebo controlled trial. *Neurology* 2002;59:1015–21.

15. Rowbotham MC, Twilling L, Davies PS, et al. Oral opioid therapy for chronic peripheral and central neuropathic pain. *N Engl J Med* 2003;348:1223–32.

16. Rowbotham MC, Reisner-Keller LA, Fields HL. Both intravenous lidocaine and morphine reduce the pain of postherpetic neuralgia. *Neurology* 1991;41:1024–8.

17. Harati Y, Gooch C, Swenson M, et al. Maintenance of the long-term effectiveness of tramadol in treatment of the pain of diabetic neuropathy. *J Diabetes Complicat* 2000;14:65–70.

18. Staahl C, Christrup LL, Andersen SD, et al. A comparative study of oxycodone and morphine in a multi-modal, tissue-differentiated experimental pain model. *Pain* 2006;123:28–36.

19. Maekawa K, Minami M, Masuda T, et al. Expression of mu- and kappa-, but not delta-, opioid receptor mRNAs is enhanced in the spinal dorsal horn of the arthritic rats. *Pain* 1996;64:365–71.

20. Zhang Q, Schaffer M, Elde R, et al. Effects of neurotoxins and hindpaw inflammation on opioid receptor immunoreactivities in dorsal root ganglia. *Neuroscience* 1998;85:281–91.

21. Dickenson AH, Kieffer B. Opiates: basic mechanism. In: McMahon SB, Koltzenburg M, Editors. *Wall and Melzack's Textbook of Pain.* London: Churchill Livingstone, 2006:427–42.

22. McLennon SM. *Persistent Pain Management*. Iowa City: University of Iowa Gerontological Nursing Interventions Research Center, Research Translation and Dissemination Core, 2005.

23. Simon LS, Lipman AG, Jacox AK, et al. *Pain in Osteoarthritis, Rheumatoid Arthritis and Juvenile Chronic Arthritis*, 2nd edn. Glenview: American Pain Society, 2002.

24. Galer BS, Coyle N, Pasternak GW, et al. Individual variability in the response to different opioids: report of five cases. *Pain* 1992;49:87–91.

25. Institute for Clinical Systems Improvement (ICSI). *Assessment and Management of Chronic Pain*. Bloomington: ICSI, 2005. Available from www.icsi.org. Accessed August 30, 2007.

26. Duhmke RM, Cornblath DD, Hollingshead JR. Tramadol for neuropathic pain. *Cochrane Database Syst Rev* 2004;(2):CD003726.

27. *Ultram ER (Tramadol Extended-Release): Prescribing Information*. Ortho-McNeil, Inc.

28. *Ultram (Tramadol): Prescribing Information*. Ortho-McNeil, Inc.

29. Hanks GW, Conno F, Cherny N, et al. Morphine and alternative opioids in cancer pain: the EAPC recommendations. *Br J Cancer* 2001;84:587–93.

30. *Avinza (Morphine Sulphate Extended-Release Capsules): Prescribing Information*. King Pharmaceuticals, Inc.

31. Neumann PB, Henriksen H, Grosman N, et al. Plasma morphine concentrations during chronic oral administration in patients with cancer pain. *Pain* 1982;13:247–52.

32. Smith MT, Watt JA, Cramond T. Morphine-3-glucuronide: A potent antagonist of morphine analgesia. *Life Sci* 1990:47:579–85.

33. Schug SA, Gandham N. Opioids: clinical use. In: McMahon SB, Koltzenburg M Editors. *Wall and Melzack's Textbook of Pain*. London: Churchill Livingstone, 2006:443–57.

34. Kalso E. Oxycodone. *J Pain Symptom Manage* 2005;29(5 Suppl.):S47–56.

35. Watson CP, Moulin D, Watt-Watson J, et al. Controlled-release oxycodone relieves neuropathic pain: a randomized controlled trial in painful diabetic neuropathy. *Pain* 2003;105:71–8.

36. Prommer E. Oxymorphone: a review. *Support Care Cancer* 2006;14:109–15.

37. Chamberlin KW, Cottle M, Neville R, et al. Oral oxymorphone for pain management. *Ann Pharmacother* 2007;41:1144–52.

38. *Opana ER (Oxymorphone HCl Extended-Release Tablets): Prescribing Information*. Endo Pharmaceuticals.

39. *Duragesic (Fentanyl Transdermal System): Prescribing Information*. Janssen Pharmaceutica Products.

40. Manfredi PL, Houde RW. Prescribing methadone, a unique analgesic. *J Support Oncol* 2003;1:216–20.

41. Trescot AM, Boswell MV, Atluri SL, et al. Opioid guidelines in the management of chronic non-cancer pain. *Pain Phys* 2006;9:1–39.

42. Ehret GB, Desmeules JA, Broers B. Methadone-associated long QT syndrome: improving pharmacotherapy for dependence on illegal opioids and lessons learned for pharmacology. *Expert Opin Drug Saf* 2007;6:289–303.

43. *Dolophine Hydrochloride (Methadone Hydrochloride Tablets): Prescribing Information*. Roxane Laboratories.

44. McNicol E, Horowicz-Mehler N, Fisk RA, et al. Management of opioid side effects in cancer-related and chronic noncancer pain: a systematic review. *J Pain* 2003;4:231–56.

45. Pappagallo M. Incidence, prevalence, and management of opioid bowel dysfunction. *Am J Surg* 2001;182(5A Suppl.):11S–18S.

46. Thomas J. Cancer-related constipation. *Am J Surg* 2001;182(5A Suppl.):11S–18S.

47. Meissner W, Schmidt U, Hartmann M, et al. Oral naloxone reverses opioid-associated constipation. *Pain* 2000;84:105–9.

48. Moore RA, McQuay HJ. Prevalence of opioid adverse events in chronic non-malignant pain: systematic review of randomised trials of oral opioids. *Arthritis Res Ther* 2005;7:R1046–51.

49. Swegle JM, Logemann C. Management of common opioid-induced adverse effects. *Am Fam Physician* 2006;74:1347–54.

50. Ballantyne JC. Opioids for chronic nonterminal pain. *South Med J* 2006;99:1245–55.

51. Mercadante S, Bruera E. Opioid switching: a systematic and critical review. *Cancer Treat Rev* 2006;32:304–15.

52. Ballantyne JC, Mao J. Opioid therapy for chronic pain. *N Engl J Med* 2003;349:1943–53.

53. Hansson P, Jensen TS, Nurmikko T, et al. EFNS guidelines on pharmacological treatment of neuropathic pain. *Eur J Neurol* 2006;13:1153–69.

54. Moulin DE, Clark AJ, Gilron I, et al. Pharmacological management of chronic neuropathic pain – consensus statement and guidelines from the Canadian Pain Society. *Pain Res Manag* 2007;12:13–21.

55. Dworkin RH, Backonja M, Rowbotham MC, et al. Advances in neuropathic pain: diagnosis, mechanisms, and treatment recommendations. *Arch Neurol* 2003;60:1524–34.

56. Oregon Health & Science University. *Patient Information Sheet.* Available from: www.ohsu.edu/ahec/pain/patientinformation.pdf. Accessed August 30, 2007.

15 • Risk management with opioids

Introduction

When used appropriately, opioids are highly effective drugs for treating chronic pain. However, both patients' and physicians' fears of drug abuse and addiction (and potential associated legal sanctions) are an important barrier to the effective use of opioids for this indication. Unfortunately, this can result in the undertreatment of pain [1,2].

The application of a standardized approach to managing chronic pain patients, referred to as 'universal precautions', is important to ensure the safe and effective use of opioids. An integral component of such precautions is the implementation of an appropriate risk management plan, including strategies to monitor, detect, manage, and report addiction or abuse.

Important definitions

Table 1 shows the definitions of addiction, physical dependence, and tolerance developed by the American Academy of Pain Medicine, the American Pain Society, and the American Society of Addiction Medicine [3].

Physical dependence
Physical dependence is defined by the occurrence of an abstinence syndrome (withdrawal) following an abrupt

Term	Description
Physical dependence	A state of adaptation that is manifested by a drug class-specific withdrawal syndrome that can be produced by abrupt cessation, rapid dose reduction, decreasing blood level of the drug, and/or administration of an antagonist
Tolerance	A state of adaptation in which exposure to a drug induces changes that result in a diminution of one or more of the drug's effects over time
Addiction	A primary, chronic, neurobiologic disease, with genetic, psychosocial, and environmental factors influencing its development and manifestations. It is characterized by behaviors that include one or more of the following: impaired control over drug use, compulsive use, continued use despite harm, and craving

Table 1. Definitions developed by the American Academy of Pain Medicine, the American Pain Society, and the American Society of Addiction Medicine.

Reproduced with permission from Elsevier (Savage SR, Joranson DE, Covington EC, et al. Definitions related to the medical use of opioids: evolution towards universal agreement. *J Pain Symptom Manage* 2003;26:655–67).

reduction of the opioid dose or the administration of an opioid antagonist [3]. An abstinence syndrome might include myalgias, abdominal cramps, diarrhea, nausea/vomiting, mydriasis, yawning, insomnia, restlessness, diaphoresis, rhinorrhea, piloerection, and chills.

Although there is extensive interindividual variability, it is prudent to assume that physical dependence will develop after an opioid has been administered repeatedly for several days. Physical dependence is not an indicator of addiction. The syndrome is self-limiting, usually lasting 3–10 days, and is not life-threatening. Opioids can be safely discontinued in physically dependent patients.

Tolerance

Tolerance ('true' analgesic tolerance or pharmacodynamic tolerance) describes the need to progressively increase the opioid dose in order to maintain the same degree of analgesia [3].

Addiction

Addiction is a chronic, neurobiological disease triggered by genetic, psychosocial, and environmental factors. It is thought to be triggered by a biologic change that leads to a protracted drive to use the drug, resulting in a preoccupation with use, craving, compulsive use, impaired control over use, or continued use despite harm [3].

Aberrant behaviors

Opioids are the second most commonly abused drugs in the US [4]. Aberrant behaviors include a wide variety of actions, ranging from those that are probably more predictive of addiction, for example [5]:

- selling prescription drugs
- prescription forgery
- stealing or borrowing another patient's drugs
- injecting oral formulations
- obtaining prescription drugs from nonmedical sources
- concurrent use of licit or illicit drugs
- multiple unsanctioned drugs escalations
- recurrent prescription losses

to those that are probably less predictive of addiction, for example [5]:

- aggressive complaining about a need for higher doses
- drug hoarding during periods of reduced symptoms
- requesting specific drugs
- acquisition of similar drugs from other medical sources
- one or two incidences of unsanctioned dose escalation
- unapproved use of drug to treat other symptoms
- reporting psychic effects not intended by the physician

Pseudoaddiction

Pseudoaddiction refers to the occurrence of problematic behaviors related to extreme anxiety associated with unrelieved pain [6]. This includes unsanctioned dose escalation, aggressive complaining about needing more drugs, and impulsive use of opioids. It can be differentiated from addiction by the disappearance of these behaviors when access to analgesic medications is increased and pain control is improved.

Pseudotolerance

Finally, pseudotolerance is the patient's perception that the drug has lost its effect. It requires a differential diagnosis of conditions that mimic 'true' analgesic tolerance. These conditions include progression or flare-up of the underlying disease, occurrence of a new pathology, increased physical activity in the setting of mechanical pain, lack of treatment adherence, pharmacokinetic tolerance, manufacturing differences of the same opioid agent, diversion, and addiction [7].

Opioid abuse and addiction

Prevalence

- The National Survey on Drug Use and Health found that past-month nonmedical use of prescription-type drugs among young adults (ages 18–25 years) increased from 5.4% in 2002 to 6.3% in 2005. This was primarily due to an increase in the use of pain relievers [8].
- In 2005, nonmedical use of hydrocodone, oxycodone, and methadone (and combinations) accounted for 51,225, 42,810, and 41,216 emergency department visits, respectively [9]. This was increased from 42,491, 36,559, and 31,874 visits in 2004 [10].

The abuse and/or diversion of prescription-controlled drugs, particularly hydrocodone and oxycodone products, therefore appears to be a growing national problem.

Screening

The physician is responsible for assessing whether the patient is at a relatively low or high risk of addiction and/or abuse. Risk factors for addiction can be divided into three categories [11]:

- psychosocial factors (eg, depression, anxiety, childhood abuse, unemployment, poverty)
- drug-related factors (eg, neuroadaptations associated with craving)

- genetic factors (eg, family history of addiction, personality disorder, pharmacokinetic genes affecting drug metabolism and transport)

The highest risk of addiction is found in a patient with characteristics from all three categories. One of the most consistent predictors of addiction is a personal or family history of substance abuse [11]. Note that this need not be a history of abuse of prescription medicines, but includes any substance (eg, alcohol).

The physician should be able to categorize questionable behaviors. For example, a patient who aggressively complains about a need for medication is more likely to have untreated distress than an addiction-related concern. On the other hand, injecting an oral formulation more likely reflects true addiction [12].

Risk assessments should be incorporated at the beginning and over the course of therapy. Tools and questionnaires can be employed to assess specific patient characteristics associated with opioid nonadherence, and for predicting aberrant drug-related behavior or addiction while receiving opioid therapy. Chabal et al. have suggested five assessment criteria for risk of drug abuse in a patient [13]:

- a focus on opioids during clinic visits
- a pattern of early refills or dose escalation
- multiple telephone calls or visits pertaining to opioid therapy
- other prescription problems
- acquisition of opioids from other sources

Other tools and questionnaires include the:

- Drug Abuse Screening Test, a 10-, 20-, or 28-item self-report questionnaire related to drug misuse [14,15]
- Pain Medication Questionnaire, a 26-item questionnaire [16]
- Screener and Opioid Assessment for Patients with Pain, a brief, self-administered screening tool for assessing the suitability of long-term opioid therapy [17]

Written agreement after detailed consent discussion
Prescribe long-acting drug without 'rescue' dose
Frequent visits and small quantities prescribed
Urine drug screen at baseline and intention to request screens in the future
Requirement that only one pharmacy will be used (with permission to contact)
Instruction to bring pill bottle to appointment (for count)
Instruction that there will be no early refills and no replacement of lost prescription without a police report documenting loss
Requirement for nonopioid therapies, including psychotherapy
Requirement for all prior records and permission to contact all other healthcare providers prior to prescribing
Requirement for referral to an addiction medicine specialist for all at-risk patients
Requirement that others be allowed to give feedback to the physician
In states with electronic prescription reporting/tracking, intention to query the database initially and regularly thereafter

Table 2. Proactive strategies in opioid prescribing.

Reproduced with permission from McGraw-Hill (Fine PG, Portenoy RK. *A Clinical Guide to Opioid Analgesia*. Minneapolis: McGraw-Hill, 2004).

- Current Opioid Misuse Measure, a 40-item questionnaire for pain patients who are already on long-term opioid therapy [18]

Avoiding and treating problematic behavior
Proactive strategies
On beginning opioid therapy, proactive strategies should be employed, based on the perceived level of risk (see **Table 2**) [19]. If problematic behavior is identified despite these strategies, the physician should reassess the patient to provide a potential diagnosis (eg, addiction, pseudoaddiction, criminal activity, depression).

Monitoring patients for adherence
Patients receiving opioids should be monitored for adherence with their treatment plan and against potential aberrant behaviors. Urine drug testing (UDT) is the most common screening method, as obtaining specimens is relatively easy and testing is affordable. In addition, the technique is well studied, has been in use for a long time, and has well-established cutoff levels and laboratory guidelines [20].

UDT can be performed to check for the presence of prescribed medications as evidence of their use, and for the presence of illicit drugs. In order to prevent stigmatization of certain patients and to ensure that no potentially nonadherent patients are missed, UDT should be applied across the board. A negative test for prescribed medications does not necessarily indicate diversion, but could be due to another reason, such as laboratory error or that the patient ran out of drugs early, either due to inadequate dosing or problematic use (ie, 'bingeing'); this result would, however, merit further discussion with the patient. The aim of UDT is not simply to ensure adherence, but to enhance the doctor–patient relationship by providing documentation of adherence to the treatment plan [21].

Pharmacotherapeutic exit strategy

On the basis of the severity of the problematic behavior, patient history, and the findings of the reassessment, the physician must make a decision regarding treatment continuation and referral (eg, to an addiction specialist). Treatment should only be continued if pain relief and maintained function are evident, control over the therapy can be reacquired, and there is improved monitoring. Any changes in the treatment plan must be comprehensively documented.

The criteria for stopping opioid therapy should be discussed with the patient prior to starting therapy, and a written exit strategy should be in place. The criteria include those of the patient [22]:

- failing to show decreased pain or increased function with opioid therapy
- experiencing unacceptable side effects or toxicity
- violating the opioid treatment agreement (see later)
- displaying aberrant drug-related behaviors

When discontinuing treatment, withdrawal symptoms can usually be avoided by using a slow opioid tapering schedule (reducing the dose by 10–20% each day) [23]. Anxiety, tachycardia, sweating, and other autonomic symptoms that persist may be lessened by slowing the taper. Clonidine at

1. Appropriate diagnosis
2. Psychological assessment, including risk of addictive disorders
3. Informed consent
4. Treatment agreement
5. Pre- or postintervention assessment of pain level and function
6. Appropriate trial of opioid therapy, with or without adjunct medication
7. Reassessment of pain score and function level
8. Regular assessment of the four As of pain medicine[a]
9. Periodic review of the pain diagnosis and comorbid conditions, including addictive disorders
10. Documentation

Table 3. Universal precautions in pain medicine [24].
[a]For a full description of the four As, see p. 209.

a dose of 0.1–0.3 mg/day over 2–3 weeks can be recommended for individuals who are known to have a history of a severe form of withdrawal.

Universal precautions

The term 'universal precautions in pain medicine' refers to a standardized approach to the assessment and management of chronic pain patients [24]. Universal precautions for opioid use are listed in the Federation of State Medical Boards' *Model Policy for the use of Controlled Substances for the Treatment of Pain*, published in 2004 [25], and in individual state guidelines.

By applying universal precautions, patient care may be improved, stigma reduced, and overall risk contained (see **Table 3**). They may also help to identify and interpret aberrant behaviors, and diagnose underlying addictive disorders where they exist. Those patients who are at risk of complicating addictive disorders can have their treatment plans adjusted accordingly. Adopting a universal precautions approach is an important step in raising the standard of care in this patient population [24].

Diagnosis

Treatable causes of pain should be identified, and therapy directed towards the cause of the pain; comorbid conditions must also be addressed.

Psychological assessment

A complete inquiry into past personal and family history of substance misuse is essential to adequately assess any patient. Patients who are using drugs (either illicit or licit, eg, alcohol) should be offered further assessment for possible substance-use disorders.

Informed consent

Informed consent is an exchange of information that protects both the physician and the patient. The physician must discuss the proposed treatment plan with the patient, including potential benefits and risks. By signing the informed consent form, the patient indicates that they understand what their physician has told them, that they willingly consent to undergoing treatment, and that they will comply with all state and federal regulations concerning the prescribing of controlled substances. A sample opioid consent form, developed and provided with the permission of the American Academy of Pain Medicine, is available from the National Pain Education Council's website at www.npecweb.org [26]. An informed consent form should be used with all patients who are receiving opioids for the treatment of chronic pain.

Opioid treatment agreements

Before the start of therapy, the expectations and obligations of both the patient and physician should be clearly established in a written or verbal agreement. The opioid agreement facilitates informed consent, patient education, and adherence to the treatment plan [27].

As a tool, the opioid agreement may also describe the treatment plan for managing pain, provide information about the side effects and risks of opioids, and establish boundaries and consequences for opioid misuse or diversion [28]. The agreement can help to reinforce the point that opioid medications must be used responsibly, and assure patients that these will be prescribed as long as they adhere to the agreed plan of care. An example opioid pain medication agreement is shown in **Figure 1** [29].

I understand that _____ (clinician name) is prescribing opioid medication to assist me in managing chronic pain. The risks, side effects, and benefits have been explained to me, and I agree to the following conditions of opioid treatment.

1. The medication must be safe and effective and help me to function better. The goal is to use the lowest dose that is both safe and effective. If my activity level or general function gets worse, the medication will be changed or discontinued by my clinician.

2. I will participate in other treatments that my clinician recommends and will be ready to taper or discontinue the opioid medication as other effective treatments become available.

3. I will take my medications exactly as prescribed and will not change the medication dosage or schedule without my clinician's approval.

4. I will keep regular appointments and will call at least 24 hours in advance if I have to reschedule.

5. *One clinician.* All opioid and other controlled drugs for pain must be prescribed by the clinician who is named above. I will not obtain medications from other clinicians or pharmacies unless I am hospitalized. I will tell any hospital or emergency room clinicians that I receive pain medications from my provider. In the event of an emergency, if I am given a prescription for pain medication, I will notify my primary clinician as soon as I am able.

6. *One pharmacy.* I will designate one pharmacy where all my prescriptions will be filled. I am responsible for prescriptions being filled on time. To avoid running out of my medications, I will contact my provider's office at least 3 business days in advance for refills. I understand that prescriptions generally will not be sent by mail or faxed.

7. I understand that lost or stolen prescriptions will not be replaced, and I will not request early refills.

8. I agree to abstain from excessive alcohol use and all illegal and recreational drug use, and will provide urine or blood specimens at the clinician's request to monitor my compliance.

9. I understand that my health information may be exchanged with other health care practitioners and pharmacists to assist in my treatment, including pain management and utilization of pain medications.

10. I understand that clinic staff (nurses, receptionists, lab staff, etc.) are very important in my success with this treatment plan. I will treat them respectfully and abide by their decisions regarding my care and the enforcement of this agreement.

11. If I am unable to follow the conditions of this agreement, I understand it may not be safe for me to continue the medication.

12. Other: _____

Patient signature:		Date:	Time:
Clinician signature:		Date:	Time:
Pharmacy:			

Figure 1. An example opioid pain medication agreement.

Pain assessment

Pain scores and function level must be recorded prior to intervention in order to assess the impact of the medication (see **Chapter 3**). Ongoing assessment and documentation of successfully met clinical goals will support the continuation of therapy, while failure to meet these goals may necessitate a change to the treatment plan.

Treatment trial

Any treatment plan must begin with a trial of therapy. Pharmacologic regimens should then be individualized according to clinical findings. The appropriate combination of agents, including opioids, nonopioids, and adjunct medications, can provide a stable therapeutic platform from which to base treatment changes.

Reassessment of pain

Regular reassessment of the patient will help document the rationale to continue or modify the current therapeutic trial. Although corroborative support from family or third parties can be useful, the patient should be the primary assessor of his/her pain (see **Chapter 3**).

The four *A*s

Reference to the four *A*s is important [30]:

- *A*nalgesia: comfort and quality of life
- *A*dverse drug effects: opioid-related
- *A*ctivity: physical and psychosocial functional status
- *A*dherence: signs of aberrant drug-related behaviors

Each time an assessment of the patient is made, it is important to specifically address each of these elements. This will help to direct therapy and support the pharmacologic decisions taken.

Review

Underlying illnesses evolve and diagnostic tests change, which means that the treatment focus may need to change over the course of time.

Documentation

Careful and complete recording of the initial evaluation and each follow-up is in the best interest of all parties. Thorough documentation, combined with an appropriate doctor–patient relationship, will reduce the potential for medical litigation and risk of regulatory sanction.

Legalities

All physicians should follow federal and state laws regarding the prescribing of controlled substances. Regarding the prescription of opioids to a reliable and clinically stable patient who is affected by a chronic disabling painful disorder, federal regulations are articulated under the Controlled Substances Act and monitored by the Drug Enforcement Administration (DEA). No specific federal requirement exists on how often a patient with chronic pain (of cancer or noncancer origin) needs to be seen at the physician's office to pick up a new prescription.

> "...What is required, in each instance where a physician issues a prescription for any controlled substance, is that the physician properly determine [that] there is a legitimate medical purpose for the patient to be prescribed that controlled substance and that the physician be acting in the usual course of professional practice...." [31].

In 2006, the DEA proposed a new rule to regulate the issuing of multiple prescriptions of controlled substances [31]. The proposal, if accepted, will "allow practitioners to provide individual patients with multiple prescriptions, to be filled sequentially, for the same schedule II controlled substance, with such multiple prescriptions having the combined effect of allowing a patient to receive over time up to a 90-day supply of that controlled substance." State guidelines and regulations vary, and physicians are required to check with their own state health departments about prescription practices and comply with those regulations. Where federal and state laws differ, the physician should follow the more stringent rule.

The undertreatment of chronic pain remains a serious problem. Physicians should not be deterred from prescribing opioids to chronic pain patients, but should ensure that appropriate risk management measures are instituted. Thorough documentation throughout the patient's care is key.

Summary

Prescription opioids have substantially and safely improved the quality of life of many patients with pain. However, opioid analgesics are also abused. By adopting regular monitoring, providing patient education, discussing benefits and risks, and establishing a formalized agreement between the physician and the patient, the likelihood of opioid abuse can be reduced while also better managing the patient's pain. **Table 4** presents a *vade mecum* for opioid therapy in chronic noncancer pain [32].

References

1. Heit HA. Addiction, physical dependence, and tolerance: precise definitions to help clinicians evaluate and treat chronic pain patients. *J Pain Palliat Care Pharmacother* 2003;17:15–29.

2. Choiniere M, Melzack R, Girard N, et al. Comparisons between patients' and nurses' assessment of pain and medication efficacy in severe burn injuries. *Pain* 1990;40:143–52.

3. Savage SR, Joranson DE, Covington EC, et al. Definitions related to the medical use of opioids: evolution towards universal agreement. *J Pain Symptom Manage* 2003;26:655–67.

4. Wilson JF. Strategies to stop abuse of prescribed opioid drugs. *Ann Intern Med* 2007;146:897–900.

5. Katz, NP. *Patient Level Opioid Risk Management. A Supplement to the PainEDU.org Manual.* Newton: Inflexxion, 2007.

6. Weissman DE, Haddox JD. Opioid pseudoaddiction – an iatrogenic syndrome. *Pain* 1989;36:363–6.

7. Pappagallo M. The concept of pseudotolerance to opioids. *J Pharm Care Pain Symptom Control* 1998;6;95–8.

8. *National Survey On Drug Use and Health 2005.* Available from: www.oas.samhsa.gov/nsduhLatest.htm. Accessed August 30, 2007.

9. Drug Abuse Warning Network, 2005. *National Estimates of Drug-Related Emergency Department Visits.* US Department of Health and Human Services, 2005. Available from: http://dawninfo.samhsa.gov/. Accessed August 30, 2007.

10. Drug Abuse Warning Network, 2004. *National Estimates of Drug-Related Emergency Department Visits.* US Department of Health and Human Services, 2004. Available from: http://dawninfo.samhsa.gov/. Accessed August 30, 2007.

Physician *vade mecum* for opioid therapy

Step 1. Therapeutic indications for initiating opioid treatment

Need for aggressive intervention, for rapid relief of moderate to severe disabling pain

Failure of nonopioid therapies; persistent pain despite reasonable trials of standard therapies, eg, nonopioid analgesics and adjuvants, physical therapy

Toxicity from nonopioid analgesics

Patient characteristics contraindicate the use of other analgesics

Step 2a. Comprehensive assessment and treatment plan

Define the medical diagnosis and identify potential treatments for the underlying disease

Assess pain intensity and the patient's level of function

Assess sleep, mood, work status, and psychosocial history

Obtain diagnostic studies and obtain appropriate consultations

Step 2b. Dealing with the high-risk or complex patient

If the patient shows 'red flags' for a substance abuse disorder (eg, conviction for a drug-related crime, history or current use of illicit drugs, regular contact with high-risk groups) then consider referral to an addiction specialist and to a pain specialist

In the meantime, consider alternative pain management strategies, such as adjuvant analgesics, nonpharmacologic and complementary medicine modalities

Step 3. Initiation of opioid therapy: patient education

Educate patient/family/caregiver:

• Use educational material on opioid therapy

• Explain definitions of tolerance, physical dependence, and addiction

• Consider a treatment agreement/informed consent form as an aid for education and documentation, and to outline procedures on form refills, dose adjustments, and emergency issues

• Discuss and document unacceptable drug-taking and drug-seeking behaviors. Discuss grounds for tapering or discontinuation

• Set realistic goals and reach agreement with the patient. Opioids are one modality in a multifaceted treatment approach

Step 4. Initiation of opioid therapy: set treatment goals

Reasonable goals include:

• clinically significant pain relief (eg, 30–50% pain relief or a 2-point reduction on a numeric scale, where 0 = no pain and 10 = the worst pain imaginable)

• an improvement in selected areas of function

• an improvement in mood or sleep

Decide whether to start a short-acting opioid analgesic or a low dose of a long-acting opioid analgesic, with or without fast-acting 'rescue' doses if breakthrough pain occurs

Consider cost, tolerability, ease of administration, and patient compliance

Step 5. Titration and maintenance

Titrate a daily opioid dose to optimal effect

Manage side effects aggressively

Periodically reassess the patient's status for the four As

Reassess treatment goals and obtain appropriate consultations and diagnostic studies

Reassessment should be ongoing to:

- guide optimal pain management

- decide whether continuation, modification, or discontinuation is required

Continue opioid therapy if the patient reports one or both of:

- pain relief

- improvement in selected areas of function and/or psychosocial functioning

Always consider opioid rotation

Recognize and manage withdrawal, tolerance, pseudotolerance, abnormal behaviors, addiction, and pseudoaddiction

Common failure criteria include:

- lack of clinically significant pain reduction

- persistent intolerable side effects

- persistent noncompliance

- rapid and intractable tolerance

- worsening of function or lack of improvement

Documentation of lack of pain reduction and lack of functional improvement serves to emphasize criteria and the need for tapering of the agent

Documentation is essential

Step 6. Occurrence of abnormal drug-taking or drug-seeking behaviors

Recognize, manage, conduct a differential diagnosis, and document

Differential diagnosis includes abnormal behaviors secondary to pseudoaddiction, pseudotolerance, and a psychiatric diagnosis (eg, encephalopathy, borderline personality disorder, depression, anxiety), as well as addiction and drug diversion

Distinguish between abandoning opioid therapy, abandoning pain management, and abandoning the patient

Table 4. *Vade mecum* for opioid therapy in chronic noncancer pain.

Coluzzi F, Pappagallo M. Opioid therapy for chronic noncancer pain: practice guidelines for initiation and maintenance of therapy. *Minerva Anestesiol* 2005;71:425–33.

11. Ballantyne JC. Opioid analgesia: perspectives on right use and utility. *Pain Physician* 2007;10:479–91.

12. Passik SD, Kirsh KL. Managing pain in patients with aberrant drug-taking behaviors. *J Support Oncol* 2005;3:83–6.

13. Chabal C, Erjavec MK, Jacobson L, et al. Prescription opiate abuse in chronic pain patients: clinical criteria, incidence, and predictors. *Clin J Pain* 1997;13:150–5.

14. Skinner HA. The Drug Abuse Screening Test. *Addict Behav* 1982;7:363–71.

15. Yudko E, Lozhkina O, Fouts A. A comprehensive review of the psychometric properties of the Drug Abuse Screening Test. *J Subst Abuse Treat* 2007;32:189–98.

16. Adams LL, Gatchel RJ, Robinson RC, et al. Development of a self-report screening instrument for assessing potential opioid medication misuse in chronic pain patients. *J Pain Symptom Manage* 2004;27:440–59.

17. Akbik H, Butler SF, Budman SH, et al. Validation and clinical application of the Screener and Opioid Assessment for Patients with Pain (SOAPP). *J Pain Symptom Manage* 2006;32:287–93.

18. Butler SF, Budman SH, Fernandez KC, et al. Development and validation of the Current Opioid Misuse Measure. *Pain* 2007;130:144–56.

19. Fine PG, Portenoy RK. *A Clinical Guide to Opioid Analgesia*. Minneapolis: McGraw-Hill, 2004.

20. Drug testing as a tool. In: Batki SL, Kauffman JF, Marion I, et al., for the Center for Substance Abuse Treatment (CSAT). *Medication-Assisted Treatment for Opioid Addiction in Opioid Treatment Programs*. Rockville: Substance Abuse and Mental Health Services Administration, 2005:143–59.

21. Heit HA, Gourlay DL. Urine drug testing in pain medicine. *J Pain Symptom Manage* 2004;27:260–7.

22. Gallagher R. Opioids in chronic pain management: Navigating the clinical and regulatory challenges. *J Fam Pract* 2004;53(Suppl.):S23–S32.

23. American Pain Society. *Principles of Analgesic Use in the Treatment of Acute Pain and Cancer Pain*, 5th edn. Glenview: American Pain Society; 2003.

24. Gourlay D, Heit HA, Almahrezi A. Universal precautions in pain medicine: a rational approach to the treatment of chronic pain. *Pain Med* 2005;6:107–112.

25. *Model Policy for the use of Controlled Substances for the Treatment of Pain*. Federation of State Medical Boards of the United States, Inc., 2004. Available from: www.fsmb.org/pdf/2004_grpol_controlled_substances.pdf. Accessed August 30, 2007.

26. American Academy of Pain Medicine. *Consent for Chronic Opioid Therapy*. Available from www.npecweb.org. Accessed August 30, 2007.

27. American Academy of Pain Management, American Pain Society. *The Use of Opioids for the Treatment of Chronic Pain. Position Statement, 2006*. Available from: www.ampainsoc.org. Accessed August 30, 2007.

28. Heit HA. *Creating and Implementing Opioid Agreements*. Available from: www.jcaremanagement.com/html/pain__creating_and_implementin.html. Accessed August 30, 2007.

29. University of Wisconsin Hospital and Clinics. *Opioid Pain Medication Agreement*. Available from www.ampainsoc.org. Accessed August 30, 2007.

30. Passik SD, Weinreb HJ. Managing chronic nonmalignant pain: overcoming obstacles to the use of opioids. *Adv Ther* 2000;17:70–83.

31. US Office of Diversion Control. *Rules – 2006*. Available from: www.deadiversion.usdoj.gov/fed_regs/rules/2006/fr0906.htm. Accessed August 30, 2007.

32. Coluzzi F, Pappagallo M. Opioid therapy for chronic noncancer pain: practice guidelines for initiation and maintenance of therapy. *Minerva Anestesiol* 2005;71:425–33.

16 • Interventional procedures and neurostimulatory techniques for pain control

Steroid injections

There is abundant evidence to associate pain syndromes (eg, radicular and axial pain) with inflammatory mediators, and also to support the role of steroids as potent anti-inflammatories in the management of pain syndromes (eg, low back pain [LBP]).

As part of a pain management program, steroids can be injected into the spine for back pain, into individual painful joints, or into areas of localized musculoskeletal pain (eg, bursitis, peritendinitis).

Epidural (extradural) injection

LBP can arise from inflammation of the spinal nerves following prolonged compression (eg, herniated disc) [1]. To relieve the pain, steroids are injected into the epidural space close to the nerve roots, normally by a pain specialist or radiologist. The number of injections is usually limited to three in 1 year in order to avoid local and systemic steroid side effects [1].

Epidural spinal injections (ESIs) to treat LBP are not new; their use has been documented since 1901 [2]. However, the use of ESIs has increased dramatically in recent years. In the Medicare population alone, there was a 271% increase in claims for lumbar ESIs between 1994 and 2001 [3]. In total, 40% of all

ESIs were associated with sciatica, radiculopathy, or a herniated disc; axial LBP diagnoses accounted for 36%, and spinal stenosis for 23%.

How effective are epidural injections?

For a treatment that has been in use for so many years, positive evidence supporting efficacy is surprisingly insufficient.

Abdi et al. recently published a systematic review of the use of ESIs in managing chronic spinal pain [4]. They divided injections into interlaminar (13 randomized trials), transforaminal (seven randomized, eight prospective, and seven retrospective trials), and caudal (eight randomized and five prospective trials) types.

The primary outcome measure was pain relief. Short-term improvement was defined as ≤6 weeks, and long-term relief as >6 weeks. The review's conclusions were as follows. For interlaminar ESIs:

- Strong evidence for short-term relief and limited evidence for long-term relief in lumbar radicular pain.
- Moderate evidence for both short- and long-term relief of cervical radiculopathy.

For transforaminal ESIs:

- Strong evidence for short-term relief and moderate evidence for long-term relief in lumbar nerve root pain.
- Moderate evidence for both short- and long-term relief in cervical nerve root pain.
- Limited evidence for relief in postlumbar laminectomy syndrome.

For caudal ESIs:

- Strong evidence for short-term relief and moderate evidence for long-term relief in lumbar radiculopathy and postlumbar laminectomy syndrome.
- Moderate evidence for short- and long-term relief in chronic LBP.

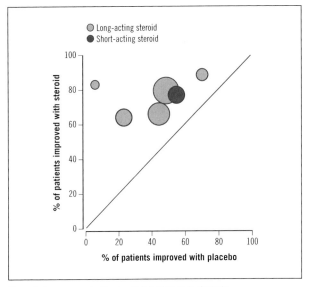

Figure 1. Improvement with steroid injection up to 2 weeks.

Reproduced with permission from Bandolier (*Steroid Injections for OA Knee*. Available from: www.jr2.ox.ac.uk/bandolier/band123/b123-3.html).

These findings, and those of other reviews and guidelines such as those from Boswell et al. [5], should be taken into account when considering ESIs as a pain management therapy.

Intra-articular injections

Steroids may also be injected into joints that are swollen and painful in order to alleviate pain. Evidence of efficacy varies. For example, injections for osteoarthritis of the knee are relatively well supported.

Godwin (2004) examined trials where intra-articular long-acting steroids (triamcinolone, methylprednisolone, and beta-methasone) were compared with placebo [6]; Arroll et al. (2004) also examined randomized trials where any formulation of steroid was compared with placebo [7].

Figure 1, combining the two studies, shows an improvement with steroid injection for up to 2 weeks. Improvement at

16–24 weeks showed a similar pattern, although with less advantage over placebo. The overall assessment is that, while the improvement is not robust, intra-articular steroid injections are helpful for alleviating painful knees in osteoarthritis, and that this is supported by clinical practice and experience [8]. In contrast, a review of steroid injections for shoulder pain (16 trials) concluded that there was insufficient evidence of benefit [9].

Maximizing benefit

- Whether an individual patient is likely to benefit from intra-articular injections is generally a specialist decision, based on clinical experience [10]. Injection for osteoarthritis of the knee has among the best support from clinical evidence, but there is a high level of placebo response.
- The procedure is generally safe. A randomized controlled trial on the safety of long-term intra-articular steroid injections reported no acute flares or infections (local or systemic) associated with the injections [11]. These results were echoed by a Cochrane review of intra-articular steroids in children and adults with rheumatoid arthritis [12].
- The steroid is commonly combined with a local anesthetic, which is injected first. The local anesthetic has the advantage of providing additional pain relief; in addition, it can help to differentiate between local and referred pain, provide fluid volume to the injection, and distribute steroids in large joints [10].
- Rifat and Moeller provide detailed advice and information about joint injection in primary care [10].

> "Clinical practice and experience suggests that intra-articular steroid injections are helpful for painful knees in osteoarthritis. The trouble is that half of the patients improved with saline alone, and the additional benefits of adding steroid were moderate" [8].

Transcutaneous electrical nerve stimulation

In this symptomatic treatment for pain, low-voltage electricity is applied to the skin via one or two pairs of electrodes. The current is delivered from a small, battery-powered unit, about the size of an MP3 player. Patients can buy or hire transcutaneous electrical nerve stimulation (TENS) machines.

TENS is delivered in three basic forms [13]:

- Conventional TENS delivers a high frequency (40–150 Hz) and low current (10–30 mA). Patients customarily apply the electrodes and leave them in place all day, turning the stimulus off for approximately 30-minute intervals during the day.
- Acupuncture-like settings deliver low-frequency stimulus trains at 1–10 Hz and high-stimulus intensity, close to the tolerance of the patient. This method is often considered for patients who do not respond to conventional TENS.
- Pulse (burst) TENS uses low-intensity stimuli firing in high-frequency bursts. No particular advantage has been established for this method.

Efficacy

TENS has been used and recommended in a wide range of conditions, but there is continuing debate in many areas of application, if not in all, about whether the treatment is more effective than placebo. When initially using a TENS machine, it is important that the patient receives detailed instruction and testing. The patient must also attend regular follow-up visits to ensure correct use of the equipment and to maximize its efficacy.

- McQuay and Moore (1996) examined the use of TENS in chronic pain. They failed to find convincing evidence that the treatment provides effective pain relief. Further trials were recommended [14].
- This was echoed 4 years later by a Cochrane review (2000) on the same subject [15].

- A separate Cochrane review (2005) found only two eligible randomized controlled trials of TENS on chronic LBP [16]. In one, TENS produced significantly greater pain relief than the placebo control. In the other, however, there were no statistically significant differences between treatment and control groups for multiple outcome measures. Again, the reviewers called for larger trials.
- Osiri et al. (2005) analyzed seven trials of TENS in osteoarthritis of the knee. Compared with placebo, TENS was found to be effective for pain control. Larger, well-designed studies are required to confirm the treatment's efficacy [17].

Risks and side effects
TENS is generally safe and well tolerated [13].

- Skin irritation and redness are the most common side effects, occurring in about one-third of patients.
- Burns can occur with excessive use, particularly if TENS is used in skin areas with decreased sensitivity.

Contraindications
TENS is contraindicated in [13]:

- patients with a pacemaker
- pregnant women (risk of premature labor)

It should also not be applied:

- over the carotid sinuses (risk of vasovagal reflex)
- over the anterior neck (risk of laryngospasm)

Peripheral nerve blocks

Peripheral nerve blocks with local anesthetics can be used as a diagnostic tool as well as a treatment modality [18]. In general, a combination of local anesthetics and steroids is used to provide patients with potentially prolonged pain relief. Blocks are performed on the peripheral nerves that are thought to be the likely pain generators for the most common pain disorders.

The following are examples of diagnostic nerve blocks.

Occipital nerve block

The *greater* and *lesser occipital nerves* supply the posterior–superior aspects of the head. The greater occipital nerve originates as a medial branch of the C2 nerve root; the lesser occipital nerve may have some innervations from the communicating branch of the C3 nerve root. The chronic pain condition originating from this nerve is called *occipital neuralgia* [19].

Ilioinguinal and genitofemoral nerve blocks

The *ilioinguinal nerve* originates from the first lumbar root. The nerve emerges from the lateral border of the psoas major muscle and makes its way to the inguinal canal, just below the spermatic cord [20]. The genitofemoral nerve, its genital branch, enters the inguinal canal and supplies the scrotal skin and the cremaster muscle.

Ilioinguinal and genitofemoral neuralgias have a variety of causes, but are often seen after surgical interventions such as inguinal herniorrhaphy [21].

Lateral femoral cutaneous nerve block

The *lateral cutaneous* is a sensory nerve that originates from the second and third lumbar roots [22]. The chronic pain from the lateral femoral cutaneous nerve is better known as *meralgia paresthetica*. Although its etiology is not clear, it seems that a significant impact on pain is due to mechanical irritation of this nerve.

Stellate ganglion block

The *stellate ganglion* is usually composed of the inferior cervical and first thoracic ganglion [23]. It is located between the C7 and T1 vertebral levels. The procedure blocks the activity of the sympathetic nerve fibers supplying the ipsilateral upper extremity and the face. Besides a diagnostic–therapeutic purpose in patients with sympathetically maintained pain, the stellate ganglion block is used for the treatment of Raynaud's disease and other conditions that cause impaired circulation to the arm.

Lumbar sympathetic block
Lumbar sympathetic block is equivalent to a stellate ganglion block for lower extremity pain. It serves a diagnostic–therapeutic role for lower extremity sympathetically maintained pain. The lumbar sympathetic chain is blocked at the L3 or L2 level in the anterolateral portion of the vertebral body [24].

Facet joint blocks and radiofrequency lesioning

A growing body of evidence shows that facet joint disease affects a significant number of people with neck and back pain. Pain elicited on neck or back extension, and radiation patterns (not below the elbow or below the knee) suggest facet joint pain. Studies have shown that cervical facet joint pain has a prevalence of 54–60%, whereas lumbar facet joints cause pain in only 15–45% of patients with chronic LBP [25].

The best diagnostic test for facet joint pain is the *block* of the medial branch of the posterior ramus of the spinal nerve. The purpose of this is to block the nerve supply to the facet joints [26].

It is likely that a subgroup of patients with cervical facet disease suffer from occipital headaches [27]. In this case, diagnostic medial branch blocks of the cervical facets should provide adequate pain relief.

Radiofrequency lesioning or denervation of the facet joints was first performed in the 1970s [28]. This technique involves the placement of a special needle under fluoroscopic guidance in a similar fashion to the placement of needles for the diagnostic block of the medial branch.

A small amount (0.5 cc) of local anesthetic is then placed at each target site. At this point, heating at 80°C/176°F for

90 seconds is performed at each level [29]. For the first 2–3 days after the procedure, the patient may experience an increase in pain; then, the patient should experience pain relief.

Discogenic pain and provocative discography

Most patients present with LBP that is limited to the back area (axial pain), or with radiation to one or both lower extremities [30]. Pain is increased by prolonged sitting or standing. On physical examination, including the straight leg raising test, the patient can appear normal.

Provocative discography is commonly used in the diagnosis of discogenic pain. During discography, needles are placed into the suspected disc (pain generator) and in two control discs under fluoroscopic guidance [31]. The contrast media is then injected into one disc at a time, with the patient blinded to the timing of the injection. The discography is positive when concordant pain is produced with injection.

Concordant pain is sought with <30 pounds per square inch above the opening pressure or <1.25 cc of contrast administered into the disc. Under these conditions the LBP that is triggered by the injection, and that corresponds to the pain familiar to the patient, is considered to be discogenic in origin.

Disc disruption and leakage of dye through the annular tear is usually seen with the onset of pain. Disc disruption alone, without reproduction of the patient's pain, is an insufficient finding for the diagnosis of discogenic pain.

There are several treatment options for a patient who presents with discogenic pain [32]. Conservative therapy, such as dynamic lumbar stabilization exercises, is helpful for some patients. Interventions include a variety of percutaneous intradiscal ablative radiofrequency procedures or, as a last resort, spinal fusion.

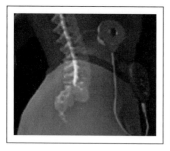

Figure 2. Spinal cord stimulation with implanted electrodes.

Reproduced with permission from Capitol Spine & Pain Centers (*Spinal Cord Stimulation*. Available from: www.treatingpain.com/pages/int_pain/spinalcordstim.html).

Spinal cord stimulation

The first reports of spinal cord stimulation (SCS) were published 30 years ago, and more recent studies have confirmed that the treatment has clinical potential [33].

SCS has been utilized for a variety of pain conditions, the most common being complex regional pain syndrome type 1, failed back surgery syndrome (FBSS), peripheral vascular disease, and angina [34]. SCS is particularly indicated with any type of neuropathic pain. Its indications have been extended to include the treatment of intractable pain due to other causes, such as cervical neuritis pain, spinal cord injury pain, postherpetic neuralgia, neurogenic thoracic outlet syndrome, and temporomandibular joint syndrome refractory to multiple surgical interventions. SCS has also been used successfully in patients with severe limb pain that does not respond to conventional methods [35].

Although a large body of work has been published, the exact mechanism of action for SCS remains unclear. SCS is achieved either percutaneously using a wire electrode threaded into the epidural space at the appropriate level (see **Figure 2**), or by laminectomy or laminotomy to suture a plate electrode to the dura [33].

Electrical stimulation currently consists of rectangular pulses delivered to the epidural space through implanted electrodes via either a constant voltage or a constant current system. Two types of system are available: a completely implantable pulse generator and a radiofrequency-coupled pulse generator with an implantable receiver.

The general experience is that, in properly selected patients, SCS will produce at least 50% pain relief in 50–60% of implanted patients. Kumar et al. have retrospectively reviewed a 15-year experience with SCS, with a mean follow-up period of 5.5 years (n=235) [36]. In their series, 59% of patients experienced satisfactory relief on follow-up; 47 patients were gainfully employed, compared with 22 patients before SCS.

Kumar reported that the results were better in patients with FBSS, complex regional pain syndrome, and peripheral vascular disease of the lower limbs; patients with cauda equina injury, phantom pain, and spinal cord injury pain did not respond as well. He also noted better results with multipolar systems. A shorter time to implantation predicted a better outcome, particularly in patients with FBSS.

Patient selection is a specialized area, and SCS is currently expensive. However, it is possible that, by reducing the overall demand for medical care, it will be cost effective in the long term.

Implantable devices for neuraxial analgesia

Intrathecal pumps

Intrathecal pumps (IPs) have recently become available for the treatment of cancer and noncancer chronic pain that responds poorly to standard pharmacologic and conservative therapeutic modalities [37]. IPs are used to deliver a variety of agents (eg, opioids, clonidine, local anesthetics, ziconotide, baclofen) into the cerebrospinal fluid.

Clinical experience and several reports indicate that clonidine and/or bupivacaine administered intrathecally can potentiate opioid analgesia for neuropathic pain. Morphine is currently the only opioid that is approved by the Food and Drug Administration for intrathecal administration, and intrathecal morphine is currently the most commonly used analgesic administered via an IP. However, treatment trials must show that the patient's pain is somewhat responsive to opioids before implantation of a morphine IP is considered [38].

A combination of an intrathecal opioid and bupivacaine enhances the effectiveness of the analgesic regimen and reduces the need for ablative or neurolytic techniques for cancer pain, particularly visceral and pelvic pain. The IP can be implanted permanently if trials are successful [38].

Intraspinally implanted tunneled catheters

Intraspinally (eg, epidurally or intrathecally) implanted tunneled catheters are being used for the temporary administration of opioids and/or local anesthetics. Neuraxial analgesia through implanted tunneled catheters can be considered in patients with advanced oncologic disease and pain that is intractable to standard interventions.

This system can provide a safe, reliable means of long-term administration of drugs into the epidural space. However, successful pain management through an intraspinal tunneled catheter system requires:

- careful education of the patient and caregiver
- repeated follow-up with pain assessment and monitoring of side effects
- close interaction between the patient, caregiver, pharmacist, home-care nurse, and physician

Neurolytic procedures for cancer pain

Neurolytic blockade can be efficacious for visceral pain in cancer; however, it is usually reserved for patients with a short life expectancy and well-localized pain syndromes. Nerve blocks that are specific for visceral pain lack durability; in some cases, they have an analgesic benefit of ≤6 months. Neurolytic blocks are primarily viewed as adjuvant therapy, and not as replacing systemic pharmacotherapy for cancer pain. Alcohol and phenol are the most widely used agents [39].

Neurolytic block of the celiac plexus

Celiac plexus blockade is well described in the literature, and it has been successfully used in the treatment of visceral pain from pancreatic cancer and upper abdominal malignancies [40].

Neurolysis of the superior hypogastric plexus

Neurolysis of the superior hypogastric plexus has been used for the treatment of visceral pain from cancer of the lower abdomen and pelvis, including gynecologic, colorectal, and genitourinary malignancies [41].

Neurolysis of the ganglion impar

Neurolysis of the ganglion impar is used for intractable rectal and perineal pain in patients who often suffer from urgency. The ganglion is located at the sacrococcygeal junction [41].

References

1. Zloczover G. *Epidural Steroid Injections and Low Back Pain*. Available from: www.spineuniverse.com. Accessed July 24, 2007.

2. Singh V, Manchikanti L. Role of caudal epidural injections in the management of chronic low back pain. *Pain Physician* 2002;5:133–48.

3. Friedly J, Chan L, Deyo R. Increases in lumbosacral injections in the Medicare population: 1994 to 2001. *Spine* 2007;32:1754–60.

4. Abdi S, Datta S, Trescot AM, et al. Epidural steroids in the management of chronic spinal pain: a systematic review. *Pain Physician* 2007;10:185–212.

5. Boswell MV, Trescot AM, Datta S, et al. Interventional techniques: evidence-based practice guidelines in the management of chronic spinal pain. *Pain Physician* 2007;10:7–111.

6. Godwin M, Dawes M. Intra-articular steroid injections for painful knees. Systematic review with meta-analysis. *Can Fam Physician* 2004;50:241–8.

7. Arroll B, Goodyear-Smith F. Corticosteroid injections for osteoarthritis of the knee: meta-analysis. *BMJ* 2004;328:869.

8. Bandolier. *Steroid Injections for OA Knee*. May 2004. Available from: www.jr2.ox.ac.uk/bandolier/band123/b123-3.html. Accessed August 1, 2007.

9. van der Heijden CJ, van der Windt DA, Kleijnen J, et al. Steroid injections for shoulder disorders: a systematic review of randomized clinical trials. *Br J Gen Pract* 1996;46:309–16.

10. Rifat SF, Moeller JL. Basics of joint injection. General techniques and tips for safe, effective use. *Postgrad Med* 2001;109:157–60,165–6.

11. Raynauld JP, Buckland-Wright C, Ward R, et al. Safety and efficacy of long-term intraarticular steroid injections in osteoarthritis of the knee: a randomized, double-blind, placebo-controlled trial. *Arthritis Rheum* 2003;48:370–7.

12. Wallen M, Gillies D. Intra-articular steroids and splints/rest for children with juvenile idiopathic arthritis and adults with rheumatoid arthritis. *Cochrane Database Syst Rev* 2006;(1):CD002824.

13. Kaye V, Brandstater ME. *Transcutaneous Electrical Nerve Stimulation*. Available from: www.emedicine.com. Accessed August 10, 2007.

14. McQuay HJ, Moore RA. *An Evidence-based Resource for Pain Relief*. New York: Oxford University Press, 1998.

15. Carroll D, Moore RA, McQuay HJ, et al. Transcutaneous electrical nerve stimulation (TENS) for chronic pain. *Cochrane Database Syst Rev* 2001;(3):CD003222.

16. Khadilkar A, Milne S, Brosseau L, et al. Transcutaneous electrical nerve stimulation (TENS) for chronic low-back pain. *Cochrane Database Syst Rev* 2005;(3):CD003008.

17. Osiri M, Brosseau L, McGowan J, et al. Transcutaneous electrical nerve stimulation for knee osteoarthritis. *Cochrane Database Syst Rev* 2000;(4):CD002823.

18. Datta S, Everett CR, Trescot AM, et al. An updated systematic review of the diagnostic utility of selective nerve root blocks. *Pain Physician* 2007;10:113–28.

19. Trescot AM. Headache management in an investigational pain practice. *Pain Physician* 2000;3:197–200.

20. Uzmansel D, Aktekin M, Kara A. Multiple variations of the nerves arising form the lumbar plexus. *Neuroanatomy* 2006;5:37–9.

21. Starling JR, Harms BA, Schroeder ME, et al. Diagnosis and treatment of genitofemoral and ilioinguinal entrapment neuralgia. *Surgery* 1987;102:581–6.

22. Windsor, RE, Thampi S. Migrating opiate pump: atypical cause of meralgia paresthetica. *Pain Physician* 2003;6:495–7.

23. Abdi S, Zhou Y, Patel N, et al. A new and easy technique to block the stellate ganglion. *Pain Physician* 2004;7:327–31.

24. Datta S, Pai U. Paradiscal extraforaminal technique for lumbar sympathetic block: report of a proposed new technique utilizing a cadaver study. *Pain Physician* 2004;7:53–7.

25. Manchikanti L, Singh V, Pampati V, et al. Is there correlation of facet joint pain in lumbar and cervical spine? An evaluation of prevalence in combined low back and neck pain. *Pain Physician* 2002;5:365–71.

26. Boswell MV, Colson JD, Sehgal N, et al. A systematic review of therapeutic facet joint interventions in chronic spinal pain. *Pain Physician* 2007;10:229–53.

27. Barna S, Hashmi M. Occipital neuralgia. *Pain Management Rounds*, 2004. Available from: www.painmanagementrounds.org. Accessed August 1, 2007.

28. Royal MA, Bhakta B, Gunyea I, et al. Radiofrequency neurolysis for facet arthropathy: a retrospective case series and review of the literature. *Pain Practice* 2002;2:47–52.

29. Brewer RP, Rho RH, Lamer TJ. The efficacy of radiofrequency lumbar facet denervation in elderly patients with mechanical low back pain. *Reg Anesth Pain Med* 2001;26(2 Suppl.):95.

30. Thomas SA. *Facet Joints and Low Back Pain*. Available from: www.spineuniverse.com. Accessed July 26, 2007.

31. Derby R. *Provocative Discography*. Available from: www.spineuniverse.com. Accessed July 31, 2007.

32. Verkuilen PE. *Lumbar Degenerative Disc Disease*. Available from: www.neurospinewi.com. Accessed July 31, 2007.

33. Stojanovic MP, Abdi S. Spinal cord stimulation. *Pain Physician* 2002;5:156–66.

34. Lee AW, Pilitsis JG. Spinal cord stimulation: indications and outcomes. *Neurosurg Focus* 2006;21:E3.

35. de Andrés J, Tatay J, Revert A, et al. The beneficial effect of spinal cord stimulation in a patient with severe cerebral ischemia and upper extremity ischemic pain. *Pain Pract* 2007;7:135–42.

36. Kumar K, Toth C, Nath RK, et al. Epidural spinal cord stimulation for treatment of chronic pain – some predictors of success. A 15-year experience. *Surg Neurol* 1998;50:110–21.

37. Knight KH, Brand FM, Mchaourab AS, et al. Implantable intrathecal pumps for chronic pain: highlights and updates. *Croat Med J* 2007;48:22–34.

38. Stearns L, Boortz-Marx R, Du Pen S, et al. Intrathecal drug delivery for the management of cancer pain: a multidisciplinary consensus of best clinical practices. *J Support Oncol* 2005;3:399–408.

39. Rowe DS. Neurolytic techniques for pain management. *Northeast Florida Med J*, 1998. Available from: www.dcmsonline.org. Accessed August 1, 2007.

40. Wong GY, Schroeder DR, Carns PE, et al. Effect of neurolytic celiac plexus block on pain relief, quality of life, and survival in patients with unresectable pancreatic cancer. *JAMA* 2004;291:1092–9.

41. de Leon-Casasola OA. Critical evaluation of chemical neurolysis of the sympathetic axis for cancer pain. *Cancer Control* 2000;7:142–8.

17 • Complementary, nonpharmacologic treatments

Psychological management

Pain is not an isolated symptom, but comes with a range of distressing emotions, such as anxiety, depression, and fear of deterioration or death. Therefore, any pain management program is inadequate if it fails to address the patient's psychological and basic human needs. Furthermore, while there is no substitute for sensitive discussion and support, some patients will need specific treatment for major psychiatric disorders, particularly depression.

Managing depression

Not unexpectedly, a high percentage of patients with pain suffer from psychiatric comorbidities such as depression. In 2004, data from primary care centers worldwide were examined by the World Health Organization [1]. The survey found that chronic pain patients were four times more likely to suffer from a depressive disorder than pain-free patients, with a corresponding negative impact on quality of life.

Note that two simple questions have a high sensitivity for the diagnosis of depression (see **Box 1**) [2]. A positive answer to either question is an indication for further enquiry, especially regarding:

- changes in appetite or weight
- sleep disturbances
- thoughts of self-harm or suicide

> **Box 1.** The two-question test.
>
> As a quick screen, the two-question test [2] has a sensitivity of 96% (ie, it can detect depression in almost all cases). Specificity is only 57%, which means that a positive answer calls for further examination. The two questions are:
>
> 1. During the last month, have you often been bothered by feeling down, depressed, or hopeless?
> 2. During the last month, have you often been bothered by little interest or pleasure in doing things?
>
> If the patient answers "no" to both questions, the screen is negative.
>
> If the patient answers "yes" to either question, consider asking more detailed questions or using a questionnaire such as the Patient Health Questionnaire-9 [3].

> In all patients with chronic pain, depressive components should be evaluated [4].

Patients with chronic pain who suffer from depression are at high risk of suicide. Depressed patients should always be asked specifically about suicidal ideation (ie, intention to commit suicide or recurring suicidal thoughts) [4].

When assessing psychological symptoms, it is important that the physician does not appear to dismiss the patient's pain. The physician needs to acknowledge that the pain is real, whether or not there is any psychogenic element [4].

> If suicidality and/or a major depressive disorder is present in the context of chronic pain, obtain a psychiatric consultation immediately [4].

Treatment

Many patients with pain will suffer from at least moderate depressive symptoms, and may benefit from antidepressants or from psychological measures such as cognitive behavioral therapy (CBT) (see the next section), or a combination of both.

Ask the patient to take an active role in the management of their pain; patients who take an active role experience less pain-related disability
Let the patient know you believe the pain is real and not in his/her head
Tell the patient that the pain is a complex problem and will require attention to a number of areas, eg, stress management, exercise, sleep pattern, quality of life
Prescribe time-contingent medications rather than pain medications as needed. Medications are then not contingent upon high levels of pain
Schedule visits regularly, rather than letting appointments be driven by increasing levels of pain
Reinforce well behaviors such as increased activity or exercise programs
Enlist the family to reinforce gains made towards improved functioning
Assist the patient in returning to work; do this in a stepwise fashion that is not dependent on the level of pain
Fear of movement or of pain due to movement is common in chronic pain patients. Graduated exposure or relaxation strategies may be helpful

Table 1. Cognitive behavioral therapy strategies.

Reproduced with permission from the Institute for Clinical Systems Improvement (ICSI) (*Assessment and Management of Chronic Pain*. Available from: www.icsi.org).

Where antidepressant medication is concerned, it is important to recognize that doses that are effective in the treatment of pain syndromes (eg, tricyclic antidepressants in postherpetic neuralgia) are generally lower than those effective in the treatment of depression [5]. Therefore, the dose may need to be increased.

In most patients with pain syndromes, especially those who are elderly or frail (and who are not already receiving tricyclic antidepressants), selective serotonin reuptake inhibitors represent the first choice of medication on the grounds of safety and tolerability [6].

Cognitive behavioral techniques

There is ample evidence that CBT is helpful in pain disorders, especially – but not only – where associated with depression [4,7].

"Cognitive behavioral approaches to the rehabilitation of patients with persistent and chronic pain are considered to be among the most helpful available" [4].

Patients may be referred to a psychologist or counselor for treatment, but there are many CBT techniques that can be implemented by the pain specialist (see **Table 1**) [4].

CBT in depression

The essential philosophy behind CBT is that the depression sufferer is prey to negative assumptions such as, "I am a failure," "There is no hope for me," and "My friends don't want me around." Treatment is directed at altering this belief system by various means, such as discussions, exercises, or keeping a diary. While CBT is normally provided by a trained therapist, effective programs are also available on CD-ROM and on the internet [8]. CBT can be as effective as medication [9], and it may be preferable in patients who cannot tolerate antidepressants.

CBT can be effective in patients with chronic pain who are suffering from depression [10].

CBT and other psychological treatments for pain

CBT has been used in the treatment of pain for >30 years [4]. A specified technique is rarely used in isolation, but rather as part of a pain management program, which may also include medication. Randomized controlled trials have noted efficacy in improving both function and mood, and in reducing pain and disability-related behavior, particularly in low back pain (LBP) [11,12].

There is evidence that CBT may be particularly effective in reducing pain and improving function in LBP [11,12].

The goals of psychological strategies in chronic pain are to:

- help the patient towards seeing pain as being under his/her control, rather than an uncontrollable medical symptom
- educate the patient about the mind–body relationship

An example of the latter is relaxation training, which helps patients direct their focus away from pain, reduce autonomic reactivity, and enhance a sense of self-control [13].

Note: this is an area in which definitions and categories vary considerably. The psychological measures listed next, as examples, sometimes come under the rubric of CBT and sometimes not.

Guided imagery
The patient focuses on a multisensory imaginary scene (eg, a favorite place). The therapist guides the patient through the image, substituting pleasant sensations, such as warmth and mental calm, for pain. Diaphragmatic breathing is an important part of the relaxation experience [13].

Progressive muscular relaxation
Patients are taught to alternately tense and relax individual muscle groups throughout the body [14]. Only nonpainful muscle groups are used. Muscle relaxation is often helpful in conditions that are associated with stress (eg, irritable bowel syndrome) [15].

Biofeedback
Biofeedback is a particularly effective means of teaching chronic pain patients relaxation and self-regulation of their physiological processes [13]. There are various forms of the treatment. One commonly used type of biofeedback machine picks up electrical signals from the muscles. It translates these signals into a form that the patient can detect, eg, a bleep or a flashing light. In order to relax tense muscles, the patient has to try to slow down the bleeping or flashing.

In a comparison of biofeedback with conservative treatments in 57 patients with chronic back pain and temporomandibular joint dysfunction, only the biofeedback group achieved significant improvements [16]. Biofeedback has also been found to be helpful in headache management and in other recurrent pain disorders.

Hypnosis

Hypnosis is another potentially effective way of helping chronic pain patients to achieve relaxation. The objective is to create a sense of distance from the pain in order to lessen its impact and make it more bearable. In one study, women with metastatic breast cancer who were undergoing weekly group therapy with hypnosis had significantly lower pain ratings over 1 year than a control group [17].

Exercise

Exercise programs can be beneficial in some chronic pain syndromes, especially LBP. The Institute for Clinical Systems Improvement has examined the evidence for exercise therapy. Its recommendations are summarized below [4]:

- Exercise has been shown to benefit patients with chronic LBP.
- No one type of exercise has been shown to be more effective than another. Studies have shown benefits from:
  – flexion exercises
  – extension exercises
  – isokinetic intensive machine muscle strengthening
  – group aerobic low-impact exercises
- Relatively inexpensive aerobic exercise programs may be as effective as physical therapy and muscle conditioning.
- Most patients with chronic pain are deconditioned from activity (often iatrogenically). A graded exercise program should start well within the patient's pain capacity and gradually increase in intensity.
- There is limited evidence showing the effectiveness of exercise in patients with neck and shoulder pain. Further randomized controlled trials are needed.

- Passive modalities (eg, transcutaneous electrical nerve
  stimulation, massage, acupuncture) should be limited and
  used only in combination with an active exercise program.

> "All patients with chronic pain should participate in a
> physical activity program to improve function and fitness.
> A cognitive behavioral approach with functional restoration
> may reduce pain and will improve function. Active patient
> participation in the care plan is essential" [4].

Acupuncture

Age-old and elaborate theories underlie the science of
acupuncture, but most present-day acupuncturists rely on the
concept of 'trigger points'; that is, areas of increased sensitivity
within a muscle that, following stimulation, cause a
characteristic pattern of pain in a related segment of the body
[18]. An example might be tender areas in the muscles of the
neck and shoulder that relate to various patterns of headache.

Treatment usually consists of stimulation of relevant pressure
points by the insertion of fine needles, although stimulation
may also be by manual pressure (acupressure) (see **Figure 1**).

The effects of acupuncture on pain are at least partially
explicable within a conventional pathophysiological model [19]:

- Acupuncture might stimulate inhibitory Aβ and
  Aδ fibers entering the dorsal horn of the spinal cord.
- Acupuncture can stimulate the release of
  endogenous opioids.

Efficacy

As practiced in North America, acupuncture is primarily a
treatment for benign, chronic diseases (eg, migraine) and
musculoskeletal pain and injury, in which areas it is best
proven. Randomized controlled trials have shown that
acupuncture is effective in [18,20–27]:

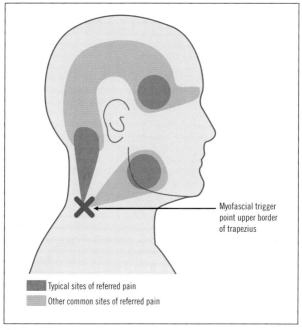

Myofascial trigger
point upper border
of trapezius

Typical sites of referred pain
Other common sites of referred pain

Figure 1. Trigger points, and their characteristic pattern of referred pain, can be treated by direct needling at the trigger point.

Reproduced with permission from BMJ Journals (Vickers A, Zollman C. ABC of complementary medicine. Acupuncture. *BMJ* 1999;319:973–6).

- migraine
- headache
- fibromyalgia
- neck pain
- LBP
- osteoarthritis of the knee
- temporomandibular joint dysfunction
- shoulder pain
- cancer-related pain

Two primary care studies are of interest:

- Vickers et al. (2004), in a randomized controlled trial, assessed the effect of acupuncture on headache (predominantly migraine) in 401 patients. The group found that the treatment leads to, "Persisting, clinically relevant benefits for primary care patients with chronic headache, particularly migraine" [28].

- Vas et al. (2004) analyzed the efficacy of acupuncture as a complementary therapy (to nonsteroidal anti-inflammatory drugs) for osteoarthritis of the knee. Forty-eight patients received acupuncture plus diclofenac, while 49 patients received placebo acupuncture (this uses retractable needles that do not perforate the skin) plus diclofenac. There were significant advantages in physical capacity and psychological functioning in the patients who received acupuncture [29].

A recent review on the efficacy of selected complementary and alternative medicine interventions for chronic pain concluded that acupuncture should be used as an adjunct in pain management for patients at risk of adverse reactions to pharmaceutical therapy, or for any patient who prefers acupuncture over drugs [30]. The review indicated that acupuncture has an efficacy level of 2–4 ('possibly efficacious' to 'efficacious') for the treatment of dental, chemotherapy-related, and premenstrual syndrome-related pain, and chronic LBP. The data were too sparse to evaluate efficacy for other chronic pain conditions. Indeed, all reviews conclude that more high-quality studies are needed.

Acupuncture has a low risk of serious adverse events [30]. The most commonly reported adverse effects are minor events such as bruising and dizziness [19].

References

1. Lépine JP, Briley M. The epidemiology of pain in depression. *Hum Psychopharmacol* 2004;19(Suppl. 1):S3–7.
2. Whooley MA, Avins AL, Miranda J, et al. Case-finding instruments for depression. Two questions are as good as many. *J Gen Intern Med* 1997;12:439–45.
3. Schwenk TL, Terrell LB, Van Harrison R, et al. *Guidelines for Clinical Care: Depression.* University of Michigan Health System, 2005.
4. Institute for Clinical Systems Improvement (ICSI). *Assessment and Management of Chronic Pain.* Bloomington: ICSI, 2005. Available from: www.icsi.org. Accessed August 7, 2007.

5.   Maizels M, McCarberg B. Antidepressants and antiepileptic drugs for chronic non-cancer pain. *Am Fam Phys* 2005;71:483–90.
6.   Chaturvedi S, Maguire P, Hopwood P. Antidepressant medications in cancer patients. *Psychooncology* 1994;3:57–60.
7.   Owen JE, Klapow JC, Hicken B, et al. Psychological interventions for cancer: review and analysis using a three-tiered outcomes model. *Psychooncology* 2001;10:218–30.
8.   Christensen H, Griffiths KM, Jorm AF. Delivering interventions for depression by using the Internet: randomised controlled trial. *BMJ* 2004;328:265.
9.   Elkin I, Shea T, Watkins JT, et al. National Institute of Mental Health Treatment of Depression Collaborative Research Program: general effectiveness of treatments. *Arch Gen Psychiatry* 1989;46:971–82.
10. Winterowd C, Beck AT, Gruener D. *Cognitive Therapy with Chronic Pain Patients.* New York: Springer Publishing, 2003.
11. Guzmán J, Esmail R, Karjalainen K, et al. Multidisciplinary rehabilitation for chronic low back pain: systematic review. *BMJ* 2001;322:1511–16.
12. Buhrman M, Fältenhag S, Ström L, et al. Controlled trial of Internet-based treatment with telephone support for chronic back pain. *Pain* 2004;111:368–77.
13. Lebovtis A. Psychological issues in the assessment and management of chronic pain. *Ann Am Psychotherap Assoc* 2002;5:19.
14. Lebovits AH, Bassman LE. Psychological aspects of chronic pain management. In: Lefkowitz A, Lebovtis AH, Woody D, et al., Editors. *A Practical Approach to Pain Management.* Boston: Little Brown, 1996:124–8.
15. Heymann-Mönnikes I, Arnold R, Florin I, et al. The combination of medical treatment plus multicomponent behavioral therapy is superior to medical treatment alone in the therapy of irritable bowel syndrome. *Am J Gastroenterol* 2000;95:981–94.
16. Flor H, Birbaumer N. Comparison of the efficacy of electromyographic biofeedback, cognitive-behavioral therapy, and conservative medical interventions on the treatment of chronic musculoskeletal pain. *J Consult Clin Psychol* 1993;61:653–8.
17. Spiegel D, Bloom J. Group therapy and hypnosis reduce metastatic breast carcinoma pain. *Psychosom Med* 1983;45:333–9.
18. Melcahrt D, Thormaehlen J, Hager S, et al. Acupuncture versus placebo versus sumatriptan for early treatment of migraine attacks: a randomised controlled trial. *J Intern Med* 2003;253:181–8.
19. Vickers A, Zollman C. Acupuncture. *BMJ* 1999;319:973–6.
20. Melchart D, Linde K, Fischer P, et al. Acupuncture for recurrent headaches: a systematic review of randomised controlled trials. *Cephalalgia* 1999;19:779–86.
21. Berman BM, Ezzo J, Hadhazy V, et al. Is acupuncture effective in the treatment of fibromyalgia? *J Fam Pract* 1999;48:213.
22. Vas J, Perea-Milla E, Méndez C, et al. Efficacy and safety of acupuncture for chronic uncomplicated neck pain: a randomised controlled study. *Pain* 2006;126:245–55.
23. Manheimer E, White A, Berman B, et al. Meta-analysis: acupuncture for low back pain. *Ann Intern Med* 2005;142:651–63.
24. Berman BM, Lao L, Langenberg P, et al. Effectiveness of acupuncture as adjective therapy in osteoarthritis of the knee: a randomised, controlled trial. *Ann Intern Med* 2004;141:901–10.
25. Smith P, Mosscrop D, Davies S, et al. The efficacy of acupuncture in the treatment of temporomandibular joint myofascial pain: a randomised controlled trial. *J Dent* 2007;35:259–67.
26. Guerra de Hoyos JA, Andrés Martín Mdel C, Bassas y Baena de Leon E, et al. Randomised trial of long term effect of acupuncture for shoulder pain. *Pain* 2004;112:289–98.
27. Mehling WE, Jacobs B, Acree M, et al. Symptom management with massage and acupuncture in postoperative cancer patients: a randomised controlled trial. *J Pain Symptom Manage* 2007;33:258–66.
28. Vickers AJ, Rees RW, Zollman CE, et al. Acupuncture for chronic headache in primary care: large, pragmatic, randomised trial. *BMJ* 2004;328:744.
29. Vas J, Méndez C, Perea-Milla E, et al. Acupuncture as a complementary therapy to the pharmacological treatment of osteoarthritis of the knee: randomised controlled trial. *BMJ* 2004;329:1216.
30. Tan G, Craine MH, Bair MJ, et al. Efficacy of selected complementary and alternative medicine interventions for chronic pain. *J Rehabil Res Dev* 2007;44:195–222.

18 • Chronic pain and insomnia

The close association between chronic painful disorders and sleep difficulties scarcely needs to be spelled out, and has been confirmed by large population studies. In a survey among 937 older people reporting arthritis, two-thirds said that sleep difficulty, not pain, was the problem for which they were most likely to consult a doctor [1]. Sleep disorder in chronic pain may also indicate an increased risk of depression and suicide [2].

> "Sleep disorders are characterized by [an] interrelationship with chronic pain such that pain leads to sleep disorders and sleep disorders increase the perception of pain. Sleep disorders in individuals with chronic pain remain under-reported, under-diagnosed, and under-treated" [3].

Some chronic pain syndromes are particularly associated with sleep problems. Examples are shown in **Table 1**, but it is to be stressed that:

- All patients with chronic pain are at increased risk of sleep difficulties, and should be asked about sleep.
- Sleep difficulties in chronic painful disease are frequently associated with emotional problems such as worry, anxiety, and depression. Patients with sleep difficulties should also be asked about mood and about specific worries.

Disorder	Potential sleep problems
Headache and migraine	Sleep disorders tend to be prevalent in more complex and severe headache patterns
	Specific headache patterns are suggestive of a potential sleep disorder (eg, morning headache, chronic daily headache)
	Treatment of sleep disorders may improve or resolve headache
Back pain	Clinical insomnia has been recorded in 53% of chronic back pain patients compared with only 3% of pain-free controls
	Affective pain ratings and health anxiety were the best predictors of insomnia severity
Osteoarthritis	75% of people attending a rheumatology clinic have reported sleep problems associated with daytime fatigue
	Restless legs syndrome is often an additional problem
Fibromyalgia	Fibromyalgia patients have been found to have significantly less sleep efficiency and non-rapid eye movement sleep, and twice as many arousals per hour of sleep compared with healthy controls
	Poor sleep quality is strongly correlated with increased symptom severity

Table 1. Pain disorders and sleep [4–7].

- All patients with a chronic pain syndrome who have evidence of depression or suicidal ideation should be referred for psychiatric assessment.

Management

There is no single effective treatment for insomnia. Management requires the careful diagnosis, assessment, and treatment of emotional disorders, effective pain control, and knowledge of cognitive behavioral interventions and pharmacologic treatments [3].

A prime necessity is to examine the patient for the presence of a depressive disorder or suicidal ideation (intention to commit suicide or recurring suicidal thoughts), both of which are frequently comorbid with pain syndromes [2]. The doctor should also consider the strong likelihood that the patient is worried about his/her disorder and its prognosis, and that he/she would welcome further discussion.

Some nonpharmacologic approaches, outlined in **Chapter 17** as treatments for depression, are also effective in sleep disturbance [3]. They include muscle relaxation, imagery training, and cognitive behavioral therapy. Aerobic exercise programs may also improve sleep; many patients with chronic pain syndromes are relatively inactive during the day. Simple sleep hygiene advice may also be helpful (see **Table 2**). Detailed advice can be found at www.rheumbook.com.

Pharmacologic therapy

Just as there is no single treatment for insomnia, there is no ideal drug. Some medication regimens have proven efficacy in some painful conditions, while others can disrupt sleep. The various options for insomnia, and their indications, are given in **Table 3**. Hypnotics, opioids, and all of the drugs commonly prescribed for insomnia should be closely monitored in patients with a history of severe sleep apnea and severe chronic obstructive pulmonary disease.

Antidepressants
- Besides being effective in the treatment of chronic pain syndromes such as postherpetic neuralgia, some antidepressants are effective for insomnia [8]. In areas such as cancer pain, improved sleep can represent a huge bonus for the patient [9].
- Some tricyclic antidepressants (eg, amitriptyline) have sedating properties and can be useful in patients with insomnia, but they can also have adverse effects. Other antidepressants, such as the selective serotonin reuptake inhibitors, have fewer side effects, but are also less sedating than the tricyclic antidepressants [8]. The sedative antidepressant trazodone may be a more effective option [10].

Subject	Advice
Evening activity	Where possible, avoid vigorous activities for 4 hours before going to bed
	Gentle exercise after that time will improve your quality of sleep
	Find an activity that calms you; spend time alone or with a family member
Food and drink	Eat a high-carbohydrate or high-fiber snack such as bread, rice, a banana, or cereal before bed – this tends to lower your core body temperature, which in turn improves sleep
	Avoid caffeine (it takes the body 10 hours to process the caffeine in one cup of coffee) and alcohol
Discomfort	If you have pain, take your medication with the snack and put on any night splints that you require
Habits	Try to go to bed at the same time each night and wake at the same time in the morning
	Do not nap for >20 minutes during the day
Rituals	Try to establish a regular ritual before going to bed
	Read something that is relaxing and takes your mind off daytime stress
	Some people find the smell of lavender soothing
Environment	Keep the bedroom slightly cooler than the rest of the house (<65°F/18°C)
	The mattress should be comfortable and firm enough for support
Getting to sleep	It is normal to take up to 30 minutes to fall asleep
	If you are lying awake for longer, get out of bed and leave the room
	Eat a healthy snack, read a book, or listen to music
	Go back to bed when you feel sleepy
Still can't sleep?	Talk to the nurse or occupational therapist on your medical team, who will be able to advise you on other ways of falling asleep
	Talk to a member of your team about any specific medical worries that you have

Table 2. Sleep hygiene: advice for patients with sleep problems [11].

Benzodiazepines and nonbenzodiazepine hypnotics

Benzodiazepines are often used to reduce the anxiety that accompanies chronic pain [8]. However, they do not have specific analgesic properties and they are associated with a

Drug	Indication
May be helpful	
Antidepressants	Given as a single nighttime dose, often the first-line choice
Long-acting opioids	Effective in chronic cancer and noncancer pain
Dopaminergic drugs	May be effective in pain associated with restless legs syndrome
Anticonvulsants (eg, gabapentin, pregabalin)	Effective in neuropathic pain (eg, postherpetic neuralgia)
May be unhelpful	
Nonsteroidal anti-inflammatory drugs	May depress slow-wave sleep and reduce restorative sleep
Neuroleptics, long-acting benzodiazepines	May impair nighttime sleep by causing daytime sedation

Table 3. Medication for insomnia in chronic pain: which drug? (Details in text.)

number of risks, such as cognitive impairment and decline in psychomotor skills, especially when combined with opioids. They should only be used for short courses [10].

Eszopiclone, zopiclone, and zaleplon, also known as non-benzodiazepine hypnotic agents, have a chemical structure unrelated to benzodiazepines. However, it appears that these drugs do interact with the γ-aminobutyric acid–benzodiazepine receptor complex, which is known to be involved in some of the pharmacologic properties of benzodiazepines, such as the sedative and anxiolytic effects [12].

Melatonin agonists

Ramelteon is a melatonin receptor agonist that has been shown to have a sleep-promoting property. Endogenous melatonin is thought to be involved in inducing the sleep-onset circadian rhythm [13]. Ramelteon should not be used in patients with hepatic impairment or in combination with fluvoxamine [14].

Opioids

Opioids may be helpful in sleep difficulties associated with both cancer and noncancer pain. Opioids such as oxycodone and methadone may be especially beneficial in pain associated with restless legs syndrome or with aching, burning, crawling, or cramping sensations. Their use may also contribute to improved daytime functioning [15].

Dopaminergic drugs

These are considered first-line for the treatment of sleep disorders associated with restless legs syndrome and associated pain in the lower limbs. Relatively long-acting formulations such as pramipexole and ropinirole are generally preferred [16].

Anticonvulsants

Anticonvulsants (eg, tiagabine, gabapentin, pregabalin) have effects that can facilitate and maintain sleep [17,18]. Gabapentin and pregabalin are particularly helpful in reducing the sleep interference of neuropathic pain disorders [18].

Adverse medications

It is important to recognize that some drugs may have adverse effects on sleep.

- Some nonsteroidal anti-inflammatory drugs, including aspirin, may depress slow-wave sleep and reduce restorative sleep [19].
- Some neuroleptic drugs (and long-acting benzodiazepines) may cause excessive daytime sedation and thus detract from refreshing nighttime sleep [20].

> "The interactions between pain states and insomnia are far-reaching. Not only is pain detrimental to sleep, mood, cognitive functioning, and behavior, but disturbances to sleep promote pain and fatigue. The relative benefits of various medications are likewise far-reaching. The ideal drug or biological substance for treating pain and sleep disorders should be relatively free of adverse side effects, should facilitate restful sleep, and should alleviate the distress of chronic disabling pain and fatigue" [20].

References

1. Jordan JM, Bernard SL, Callahan LF, et al. Self-reported arthritis-related disruptions in sleep and daily life and the use of medical, complementary, and self-care strategies for arthritis: the National Survey of Self-care and Aging. *Arch Fam Med* 2000;9:143–9.

2. Smith MT, Perlis ML, Haythornthwaite JA. Suicidal ideation in outpatients with chronic musculoskeletal pain: an exploratory study of the role of sleep onset insomnia and pain intensity. *Clin J Pain* 2004;20:111–18.

3. Stiefel F, Stagno D. Management of insomnia in patients with chronic pain conditions. *CNS Drugs* 2004;18:285–96.

4. Rains JC, Poceta JS. Sleep and headache disorders: clinical recommendations for headache management. *Headache* 2006;46(Suppl. 3):S147–8.

5. Tang NK, Wright KJ, Salkovskis PM. Prevalence and correlates of clinical insomnia co-occurring with chronic back pain. *J Sleep Res* 2007;16:85–95.

6. Pincus T, Swearingen C, Wolfe F. Toward a multidimensional Health Assessment Questionnaire (MDHAQ): assessment of advanced activities of daily living and psychological status in the patient-friendly health assessment questionnaire format. *Arthritis Rheum* 1999;42:2220–30.

7. Rizzi M, Sarzi-Puttini P, Atzeni F, et al. Cyclic alternating pattern: a new marker of sleep alteration in patients with fibromyalgia? *J Rheumatol* 2004;31:1193–9.

8. American Chronic Pain Association (ACPA). *ACPA Medications and Chronic Pain: Supplement 2007*. Rocklin: ACPA, 2007.

9. McQuay HJ, Moore RA. Antidepressants and chronic pain. *BMJ* 1997;314:763–4.

10. Institute for Clinical Systems Improvement (ICSI). *Assessment and Management of Chronic Pain*. Bloomington: ICSI; 2005. Available from: www.icsi.org. Accessed August 15, 2007.

11. Thompson A. *Sleep Hygiene*, 2005. Available from: www.rheumbook.com/rheum_info/coping_arthritis/sleep%20hygiene.html. Accessed August 15, 2006.

12. Roy-Byrne PP. The GABA-benzodiazepine receptor complex: structure, function, and role in anxiety. *J Clin Psychiatry* 2005;66(Suppl. 2):14–20.

13. Lieberman JA. Update on the safety considerations in the management of insomnia with hypnotics: incorporating modified-release formulations into primary care. *Prim Care Companion J Clin Psychiatry* 2007;9:25–31.

14. Hussar DA. New drugs: ramelteon, tipranavir, nepafenac, and deferasirox. *J Am Pharm Assoc* 2006;46:107–11.

15. Walters AS, Winkelmann J, Trenkwalder C, et al. Long-term follow-up on restless legs syndrome patients treated with opioids. *Mov Disord* 2001;16:1105–9.

16. Moldofsky H. Pain and insomnia: what every clinician should know. *Medscape Neurology & Neurosurgery* 2004;6. Available from: www.medscape.com/viewarticle/494872. Accessed August 15, 2007.

17. Todorov AA, Kolchev CB, Todorov AB. Tiagabine and gabapentin for the management of chronic pain. *Clin J Pain* 2005;21:358–61.

18. Tassone DM, Boyce E, Guyper J, et al. Pregabalin: a novel gamma-aminobutyric acid analogue in the treatment of neuropathic pain, partial onset seizures, and anxiety disorders. *Clin Ther* 2007;29:26–48.

19. Lavie P, Nahir M, Lorber M, et al. Nonsteroidal anti-inflammatory drug therapy in rheumatoid arthritis patients. Lack of association between clinical improvement and effects on sleep. *Arthritis Rheum* 1991;34:655–9.

20. Sutton DA, Moldofsky H, Badley EM. Insomnia and health problems in Canadians. *Sleep* 2001;24:665–70.

19 • Management of medication-related side effects

Many of the drug groups that are used in pain management have troublesome and/or serious side effects, which may lead to complications. Patients who are starting a course of treatment should be told what side effects to expect and when to report them to healthcare staff (eg, postural hypotension with tricyclic antidepressants [TCAs], constipation with opioids). Many of the adverse effects associated with pain medications can be prevented or minimized. In addition, the patient may develop tolerance against a number of side effects (eg, sedation with TCAs, nausea with opioids).

Table 1 summarizes the side effects associated with various drug groups and their management, based on the recommendations of the Institute for Clinical Systems Improvement [1]. The full guidance, with adult and pediatric doses, can be found at www.icsi.org.

Nonsteroidal anti-inflammatory drugs

All nonsteroidal anti-inflammatory drugs (NSAIDs) are associated with an increased risk of gastritis and of bleeding from any part of the digestive tract [1].

- A single dose of aspirin may cause gastric irritation and drowsiness [2].

Drug category	Side effect	Management
NSAIDs	GI upset	Give misoprostol
		Tell the patient to take the medication with food
		Consider antacids, H_2-antagonists, proton-pump inhibitors, switching to a COX-2 inhibitor
	Bleeding tendency	Consider trisilicate or disalcid
		NSAIDs should be immediately discontinued if there are signs of bleeding (eg, hematemesis, melena, anemia)
	Nephrotoxicity	Consider alternatives (eg, sulindac)
		Note that toxicity is dose-dependent for all NSAIDs
COX-2 inhibitors	GI upset	Consider a proton-pump inhibitor or discontinue
	Liver dysfunction	Monitor closely or discontinue
	Nephrotoxicity	Discontinue
Acetaminophen	Hepatotoxicity	Limit dose to ≤2 g/day
		Use a lower dose in pre-existing liver disease
Opioids	Nausea and vomiting	Give hydroxyzine, diphenhydramine, or ondansetron with each dose of SR opioid medication, or transdermal scopolamine during the initial opioid therapy
		Consider opioid rotation (eg, to hydromorphone or oxycodone) if nausea persists
		Nondrug treatment: toast/crackers, sherbet, pretzels, oatmeal, soft and bland fruits and vegetables
		Acupuncture/acupressure might help some patients
		Give senna/docusate, bisacodyl, milk of magnesia, magnesium citrate, or lactulose

Table 1. Complications and side effects of medications. COX: cyclooxygenase; GI: gastrointestinal; IV: intravenous; NSAID: nonsteroidal anti-inflammatory drug; PO: oral; SR: sustained release. *Continued on facing page.*

Adapted with permission from the Institute for Clinical Systems Improvement (ICSI) (*Assessment and Management of Chronic Pain*. Available from www.icsi.org).

Drug category	Side effect	Management
Opioids	Constipation	Nondrug treatment: good hydration; if PO intake: prunes, prune juice, Smooth Move Tea; mobility
	Pruritus	Give diphenhydramine
		Consider changing opioid, as above
		Give propofol or naloxone for epidural/intrathecal morphine
	Myoclonus	Give clonazepam or lorazepam; consider changing opioid, as above
	Respiratory depression	Give naloxone: Dilute 0.4 mg (1 mL) naloxone with 9 mL normal saline
		Administer 0.04 mg (1 mL) boluses IV until respiratory rate increases (onset time after an incremental dose is <2 min)
		Naloxone has a short half-life (45–90 min), so additional doses are often required. Monitor patients for return of pain and opioid toxicity, and opioid withdrawal symptoms. Monitor closely for ≥24 hours
Antidepressants	See main text	See main text
Anticonvulsants	Somnolence or cerebellar symptoms	Decrease dose
Carbamazepine	Myelosuppression	Change to another antiepileptic drug
		Note that the only indication for carbamazepine is trigeminal neuralgia, and that monitoring of serum concentrations is mandatory
Corticosteroids	Hyperglycemia	Give appropriate management
		Consider changing to an NSAID

Table 1. *Continued.*

- Use with caution in the elderly or those who are at higher risk of gastrointestinal adverse effects, or combine with the gastroprotective agent misoprostol or a proton-pump inhibitor [3].
- Diabetic patients should be monitored for signs of reduced renal function [1].

- Monitor all NSAID use, including patient use of nonprescription drugs, in order to avoid duplication of therapy and adverse effects [1].
- NSAIDs should never be used in combination with one another.
- Dosing intervals should be increased in elderly patients. A younger patient with postoperative pain could be treated with ibuprofen 800 mg three times daily, while an effective dose for a patient aged 80 years could be 200 mg twice daily. The maximum daily dose of ibuprofen is 3,200 mg/day.

> "The elderly are at special risk for NSAID toxicity and should be carefully monitored and started on the lowest recommended dose" [4].

Opioids

An opioid regimen should be managed and monitored by one prescriber [5].

- Up to two-thirds of patients suffer from nausea and vomiting when starting morphine, which can last up to 7 days. All patients should be offered an antiemetic [5].
- Constipation occurs in up to 90% of patients who are receiving opioids for noncancer pain [6]. It should be treated preventively [1], and bowel function should be monitored regularly. It is common to use both softening and stimulating laxatives [6]. Use the latter cautiously in patients who are at risk of bowel obstruction [5].
- To avoid dry mouth, patients should be encouraged to adopt good oral care, suck boiled acidic sweets, and use sugar-free chewing gum [5]. They should also be advised to take supplementary oral fluoride tablets to avoid dental caries. Contact with a dental hygienist is important.
- Urinary retention and pruritus are uncommon, but can be a problem with spinal administration of opioids [5].

"Patients with cancer often see several doctors and may receive opioids from more than one clinician. To avoid this happening, it is good practice for one person to take the lead role in prescribing" [5].

Antidepressants

Amitriptyline is the best proven antidepressant in neuropathic pain, but it has the most side effects (eg, dry mouth, drowsiness, postural hypotension) [1]. Where possible, avoid amitriptyline in elderly or frail patients and in those at cardiac risk, or start with a much reduced dose.

- Amitriptyline should be started at 10–25 mg once daily, with dose escalation of 10–25 mg/week according to pain relief and adverse effects [1]. The dose should be taken 2–3 hours before bedtime, especially where insomnia is a problem [7]. The total dose can be increased to 75–150 mg/day [1]. Doses should be far less in elderly or frail patients, where 10–20 mg/day is often adequate.
- Desipramine or doxepin may be associated with fewer side effects. However, selective serotonin reuptake inhibitors (SSRIs) are less effective than TCAs in neuropathic pain [7].
- TCAs are extremely dangerous in overdose [8]. Where possible, avoid prescribing TCAs in potentially suicidal patients, or prescribe in small quantities. It is strongly recommended that all patients with evidence of suicidal ideation be directly referred for psychiatric assessment.
- In the treatment of depression associated with chronic pain, first consider the use of nonpharmacologic interventions (eg, cognitive behavioral therapy), especially in children and adolescents [9].
- In the treatment of depression, SSRIs (eg, fluoxetine) are usually the first-line choice of medication, especially in elderly or frail patients [10].

Anticonvulsants

- Lamotrigine may be associated with severe, possibly life-threatening dermatologic side effects [11,12]. Start with a low dose and increase gradually.
- Gabapentin shows considerable variation in tolerance. The most commonly reported side effects are dizziness, somnolence, and peripheral edema [12]. Again, start with a low dose.
- Carbamazepine is contraindicated in patients with liver abnormalities, bone marrow suppression, or known sensitivity to tricyclic compounds [1].

> To minimize the risk of side effects, begin anticonvulsants at low doses and increase gradually, as needed.

References

1. Institute for Clinical Systems Improvement (ICSI). *Assessment and Management of Chronic Pain*. Bloomington: ICSI, 2005. Available from: www.icsi.org. Accessed August 30, 2007.
2. Edwards JE, Oldman A, Smith L, et al. Single dose oral aspirin for acute pain. *Cochrane Database Syst Rev* 2000;(2):CD002067.
3. Michigan Quality Improvement Consortium (MQIC). *Medical Management of Adults with Osteoarthritis*. Southfield: MQIC, 2005. Available from: www.mciq.org. Accessed August 30, 2007.
4. Wisconsin Medical Society Task Force on Pain Management. Guidelines for the assessment and management of chronic pain. *WMJ* 2004;103:13–42.
5. Quigley C. The role of opioids in cancer pain. *BMJ* 2005;331:825–9.
6. Panchal SJ, Müller-Schwefe P, Wurzelmann JI. Opioid-induced bowel dysfunction: prevalence, pathophysiology and burden. *Int J Clin Pract* 2007;61:1181–7.
7. McQuay H, Moore RA. Antidepressants and chronic pain. *BMJ* 1997;314:763–4.
8. Buckley NA, McManus PR. Fatal toxicity of serotonergic and other antidepressant drugs: analysis of United Kingdom mortality data. *BMJ* 2002;325:1332–3.
9. Eccleston C, Malleson P. Managing chronic pain in children and adolescents. *BMJ* 2003;326:1408–9.
10. Chaturvedi S, Maguire P, Hopwood P. Antidepressant medications in cancer patients. *Psychooncology* 1994;3:57–60.
11. Nurmikko TJ, Nash TP, Wiles JR. Recent advances: control of chronic pain. *BMJ* 1998;317:1438–41.
12. Maizels M, McCarberg B. Antidepressants and antiepileptic drugs for chronic noncancer pain. *Am Fam Physician* 2005;71:483–90.

Further reading

General

Benzon HT, Raja SN, Molloy RE, et al. *Essentials of Pain Medicine and Regional Anesthesia*, 2nd edn. London: Churchill Livingstone, 2004.

McMahon S, Koltzenburg M, Editors. *Wall and Melzack's Textbook of Pain*, 5th edn. London: Churchill Livingstone, 2005.

Pappagallo M, Editor. *Neurological Basis of Pain*. New York: McGraw-Hill, 2005.

National Institutes of Health. National Institute of Neurological Disorders and Stroke. *NINDS Chronic Pain Information Page*. Available from: www.ninds.nih.gov/disorders/chronic_pain/chronic_pain.htm.

International Association for the Study of Pain: www.iasp-pain.org.

Pain Control In The Primary Care Setting. Available from: www.association-office.com. (This handbook is designed for healthcare professionals as a tool to improve the quality of pain management, with particular emphasis on the primary care setting.)

Back pain

National Institutes of Health. *Back Pain*. Available from: www.nlm.nih.gov/medlineplus/backpain.html. (An information page for patients and professionals, with numerous links.)

NHS Centre for Reviews and Dissemination, University of York. Acute and chronic low back pain. *Effective Health Care* 2000;6. Available from: www.york.ac.uk/inst/crd/ehc65.pdf.

Cancer pain

Guideline for the Management of Cancer Pain in Adults and Children. Available from: www.association-office.com/ APS/etools/products/products.cfm. (A comprehensive, peer-reviewed and evidence-based book.)

Osteoarthritis

Arthritis Research Campaign. *Osteoarthritis: An Information Booklet*. Available from: www.arc.org.uk/about_arth/booklets/ 6025/6025.htm. (A comprehensive summary, primarily for patients, but also likely to be helpful to professionals, with links.)

Ischemic pain

Donnelly R, London NJM, Editors. *ABC of Arterial and Venous Disease*. London: BMJ Publishing, 2000.

Irritable bowel syndrome

Agrawal A, Whorwell PJ. Irritable bowel syndrome: diagnosis and management. *BMJ* 2006;332:280–3.

Headache

Olesen J, Tfelt-Hansen P, Welch KMA, Editors. *The Headaches*, 3rd edn. Philadelphia: Lippincott Williams & Wilkins, 2005.

Silberstein SD, Lipton RB, Goadsby PJ, et al. *Headache in Primary Care,* 1st edn. Oxford: Isis Medical Media, 1999.

International Headache Society: www.i-h-s.org.

The Headache Classification Subcommittee of the International Headache Society. The International Classification of Headache Disorders, 2nd edn. *Cephalalgia* 2004;24(Suppl. 1).

Fibromyalgia

National Institute of Arthritis and Musculoskeletal and Skin Diseases. *Fibromyalgia: Summaries of Research*, 2004. Available from: www.niams.nih.gov/ne/highlights/spotlight/2004/fibro_sum.htm.

Cognitive behavioral therapy

Beck JS. *Cognitive Therapy: Basics and Beyond*. New York: The Guildford Press, 1995.

McCracken LM, Editor. *Contextual Cognitive–Behavioral Therapy for Chronic Pain*. Seattle: International Association for the Study of Pain, 2005.

Complementary medicine

National Center for Complementary and Alternative Medicine, National Institutes of Health. *Acupuncture*. Available from: http://nccam.nih.gov/health/acupuncture/.

Index

As the subject of this book is chronic pain, entries under this subject have been kept to a minimum. Readers are advised to look under more specific terms. Page numbers in **bold** indicate figures: page numbers in *italics* refer to material in tables or boxed material.

CME questions

Answers should be completed online (instructions on p. 276) or in the space provided on the Evaluation form on p. 276.

Section 1: Physiology of pain; Epidemiology of chronic pain; Pain assessment

1. **For clinical purposes, the two main categories of pain are:**
    a. Peripheral and central nervous system pain
    b. Somatic and visceral pain
    c. Neurologic and diabetic pain
    d. Nociceptive and neuropathic pain
    e. Cancer and noncancer pain

2. **Chronic pain is:**
    a. Associated with blood pressure and body temperature changes
    b. Used by the body to signal danger or that something is wrong
    c. A long process, taking at least 1 year to manifest
    d. Caused by depression and other psychiatric disorders
    e. Associated with long-term peripheral and central nervous system pain pathway changes

3. **The processing of nociceptive pain can be broken down into the following key stages:**
    a. Transduction; transmission to the spinal cord; spinal cord processing; ascending pathways to and processing by the brain; and descending pathways
    b. Signaling; activation of N-methyl-D-aspartate receptors; release of neurotransmitters; hypersensitization; long-term changes
    c. Hyperexcitability of central neurons (central sensitization); reorganization of synaptic connectivity in the spinal cord and elsewhere in the central nervous system (central sensitization); impaired segmental and nonsegmental inhibition
    d. Peripheral sensitization; ectopic discharges; central sensitization; impaired inhibition

4. **In nociceptive pain, pain is transmitted via:**
    a. A fibers and $C\alpha$ fibers
    b. $A\delta$ fibers and B fibers
    c. $B\beta$ fibers and D fibers
    d. $A\delta$ fibers and C fibers
    e. C fibers and $D\beta$ fibers

5. **Which of the following factors are associated with chronic pain? (Select all that apply.)**
    a. Low environmental temperature
    b. Schizophrenia
    c. High social support
    d. History of injury
    e. Depression

6. **Which of the following statements is NOT correct?**
    a. Chronic pain sufferers are heavy users of healthcare services
    b. Approximately 30% of the population has experienced chronic pain
    c. There is a significant female preponderance for chronic pain
    d. Chronic pain sufferers have low scores for quality of life
    e. Pain is a natural part of growing old

7. **Chronic and recurrent pain in children and adolescents has a point prevalence of approximately:**
    a. 5%
    b. 15%
    c. 30%
    d. 50%
    e. 75%

8. **The most common pain complaint in children and adolescents is:**
    a. Toothache
    b. Abdominal pain
    c. Limb pain
    d. Headache
    e. Back pain

9. **The most reliable assessor of a patient's pain is:**
    a. The patient's primary care physician
    b. The patient's friends/relatives
    c. The patient
    d. A pain specialist

10. **A variety of well-validated pain scales are available. The physician should choose the one that is most appropriate to the patient and apply the method systematically. For which patient group would you use the Wong–Baker faces pain rating scale?**
    a. Those with cognitive impairment
    b. Children aged ≥3 years
    c. Adults with language barriers
    d. All of the above

Section 2: Low back pain syndrome; Osteoarthritis; Ischemic pain syndromes; Visceral pain syndromes

1. **Which of the following is NOT an assessment goal in the evaluation of patients with chronic low back pain?**
    a. Identify the source of the pain
    b. Conduct a segmental range of motion test
    c. Assess the degree of pain and functional limitation
    d. Define the contributing factors
    e. Develop a management strategy

2. **Which of the following are common clinical features of osteoarthritis? (Select all that apply.)**
    a. Crepitus
    b. Bony enlargement
    c. Warmth
    d. Effusion
    e. Muscle weakness

3. **Anginal pain in the neck and jaw is caused by:**
   a. Activation of the hypothalamic, reticular, and thalamic loci and the prefrontal cortex by the spinothalamic tract
   b. Release of adenosine and bradykinin
   c. Excitation of spinothalamic tract cells in the upper thoracic and lower cervical segments
   d. Excitation of the upper cervical spinothalamic tract cells by descending impulses from the nucleus tractus solitarii in the brainstem

4. **Which of the following are characteristic of pain in myocardial infarction? (Select all that apply.)**
   a. Usually lasts 5–10 minutes
   b. Relieved by rest
   c. Associated with dyspnea, sweating, nausea, or vomiting
   d. Crushing retrosternal chest pain
   e. Centralized to the chest area

5. **Which of the following is NOT a risk factor for intermittent claudication?**
   a. Caffeine
   b. Older age
   c. Diabetes
   d. Sedentary lifestyle
   e. Hypertension

6. **The three characteristics of pain in intermittent claudication are:**
   a. Cramping pain in the foot; relieved by stretching; intermittent
   b. Cramping pain in the calves; relieved by rest; reproducible
   c. Stabbing pain in the thigh; relieved by activity; sporadic
   d. Aching pain in the knee; relieved by cold; constant

7. **Sickle cell pain can be effectively managed. Which of the following statements is NOT true?**
   a. Tolerance and physical dependence are common in sickle cell patients, and opioids should be avoided
   b. Pain management should be aggressive to enable patients to maintain maximum functional ability
   c. Severe pain should be considered a medical emergency
   d. Nonsteroidal anti-inflammatory drugs should be prescribed for mild to moderate pain, unless contraindicated
   e. Pain management should be part of a comprehensive treatment plan that includes psychological, behavioral, and physical interventions

8. **It is important to look out for 'red flags' when examining a patient who presents with the symptoms of irritable bowel syndrome (IBS). Which of the following would indicate that a diagnosis other than IBS must be excluded? (Select all that apply.)**
   a. Vomiting
   b. Family history of colorectal cancer
   c. Fever
   d. High caffeine intake
   e. High emotional stress

9. **Possible causes of secondary dysmenorrhea include which of the following? (Select all that apply.)**
   a. Inflammatory bowel disease
   b. Intermittent claudication
   c. Hypertension
   d. Pelvic inflammatory disease
   e. Endometriosis

10. **There is no typical pattern of pain in chronic pelvic pain:**
    a. True
    b. False

Section 3: Neuropathic pain syndromes; Headache; Fibromyalgia; Cancer pain

1. **Patients with neuropathic pain can present with many abnormal sensory symptoms and signs. Which term does the phrase 'Pain elicited by nonnoxious stimuli' describe?**
   a. Dysesthesia
   b. Hyperalgesia
   c. Paresthesia
   d. Allodynia
   e. Hyperpathia

2. **Which of the following is NOT a differential pain diagnosis for diabetic neuropathy?**
   a. Plantar fasciitis
   b. Radiculopathy
   c. Osteoarthritis
   d. Fibromyalgia
   e. Claudication

3. **Postherpetic neuralgia (PHN) occurs in 25–50% of patients aged >50 years following herpes zoster infection. Which of the following classes of pharmacologic agents does NOT have established efficacy for PHN pain?**
   a. Benzodiazepines
   b. Gabapentinoids
   c. Opioids
   d. Topical analgesics and anesthetics
   e. Tricyclic antidepressants

4. **Complex regional pain syndrome (CRPS) can develop following a distal limb traumatic injury and subsequent limb immobilization (often an important predisposing factor in the medical history of this disorder). Which of the following are part of the International Association for the Study of Pain criteria for CRPS type 1? (Select all that apply.)**
   a. Pain that is disproportionate in severity to the inciting noxious event
   b. Edema
   c. Weight gain
   d. Comorbidities that would account for the pain
   e. Changes in skin blood flow

5. **In the headache patient, red flags can point to a serious underlying pathology, and indicate a need for referral and/or neuroimaging (CT or MRI). Which of the following is NOT a red flag in headache?**
   a. 'Thunderclap' headache
   b. Stress at home or work
   c. Focal neurologic signs or symptoms
   d. Change in existing headaches
   e. Associated systemic symptoms

6. **In the prophylaxis of cluster headaches, the first-line treatment is:**
   a. Verapamil
   b. Prednisone
   c. Oxygen and/or sumatriptan
   d. Anticonvulsants
   e. Opioids

7. **Fibromyalgia has been well reported in this country. The overall prevalence in women has been estimated at:**
   a. 0.1%
   b. 3%
   c. 9%
   d. 12%
   e. 17%

8. **The pain of fibromyalgia is often:**
   a. Described as "aching all over"
   b. Associated with numbness and tingling
   c. Found in all four quadrants of the body
   d. Associated with 'tender points'
   e. All of the above

9. **Which of the following does NOT indicate a neuropathic pain component in cancer pain?**
   a. The pain is musculoskeletal, arising from tissues such as the skin, mucosa, muscles, bones, and ligaments
   b. There are signs of sensory or motor dysfunction in the pain area
   c. Pain therapy with ordinary analgesics has been unsuccessful, or the patient requires high doses of strong opioids
   d. The pain area corresponds to the innervation territory of a nerve, nerve root, or central nervous system structure
   e. The pain is described as burning, tingling, pins and needles, electric, or stabbing

10. **Metastasis to bone is the most common cause of pain in cancer patients; the pain is often severe and debilitating. Which of the following is appropriate for severe cancer pain that is not amenable to conventional drug delivery routes?**
   a. Implantable intrathecal pump
   b. Neuroablative procedures
   c. Palliative surgery
   d. Radiation therapy
   e. All of the above

Section 4: Breakthrough pain; Nonopioid analgesics and adjuvants; Opioids; Risk management with opioids

1. **Transmucosal fentanyl is a lipophilic opioid used in breakthrough pain. Which two amounts indicate the onset of action and duration of action, respectively, of transmucosal fentanyl?**
   a. 5–10 minutes and 1–2 hours
   b. 10–15 minutes and >2 hours
   c. 20–30 minutes and 1–2 hours
   d. 20–30 minutes and >4 hours
   e. 45–60 minutes and 4–6 hours

2. **Acetaminophen has analgesic and antipyretic properties, but it can also have chronic adverse renal or hepatic effects. Therefore, acetaminophen, alone or in combination, should be limited to which dose?**
   a. <0.5 g/day
   b. <1 g/day
   c. <2 g/day
   d. <4 g/day
   e. <6 g/day

3. **Which of the following is a selective COX-2 inhibitor?**
   All of the rest are nonselective inhibitors.
   a. Celecoxib
   b. Ibuprofen
   c. Tolmetin
   d. Piroxicam
   e. Sulindac

4. **Gabapentin is a first-line treatment in:**
   a. Visceral pain
   b. Ischemic pain
   c. Low back pain
   d. Neuropathic pain
   e. Headache

5. **The adverse effects of tricyclic antidepressants include which of the following? (Select all that apply.)**
   a. Weight loss
   b. Dry mouth
   c. Sedation
   d. Urinary retention
   e. Nausea

6. **The serotonin and norepinephrine reuptake inhibitor duloxetine is FDA-approved for the treatment of which type of pain?**
   a. Postamputation pain
   b. Cancer pain
   c. Headache
   d. Sickle cell pain
   e. Pain secondary to diabetic neuropathy

7. **With regards to opioids, what is pseudotolerance?**
   a. The need to escalate the opioid dose to maintain the same analgesic effect
   b. The occurrence of problematic behaviors related to extreme anxiety associated with unrelieved pain
   c. The patient's perception that a drug has lost its effect
   d. The occurrence of withdrawal following an abrupt reduction of the opioid dose or the administration of an opioid antagonist

8. **Opioid rotation refers to the switch from one opioid to another when the degree of analgesia obtained is limited by adverse effects. Upon switching from opioid A to opioid B, by which percentage should you decrease the equianalgesic dose of opioid B?**
   a. 5–17%
   b. 10–28%
   c. 25–53%
   d. 50–67%
   e. 75–92%

9. **Which of the following is NOT a common adverse effect of chronic opioid therapy?**
   a. Nausea
   b. Constipation
   c. Drowsiness
   d. Delirium
   e. Rash

10. **Reference to the four As is important in the risk management of the chronic pain patient on opioids. Which of the following is NOT one of the four As?**
    a. Adherence
    b. Activity
    c. Analgesia
    d. Avoidance
    e. Adverse drug effects

11. **A written exit strategy is an important part of opioid therapy. The strategy should be in place before therapy begins, and both the patient and physician should be clear on the criteria for stopping opioid therapy. These criteria might include which of the following? (Select all that apply.)**
   a. The patient violates the opioid treatment agreement
   b. The patient aggressively complains about the need for higher doses
   c. The patient engages in a single episode of unsanctioned drug escalation
   d. The patient fails to show increased analgesia or improved function with opioid therapy
   e. The patient experiences unacceptable side effects or toxicity

12. **Aberrant behaviors come in a wide variety of forms. Which TWO of the following behaviors are probably MORE indicative of addiction? The others are all probably less indicative of addiction.**
   a. Requesting specific drugs
   b. Unapproved use of drug to treat other symptoms
   c. Drug hoarding during periods of reduced symptoms
   d. Injecting oral formulations
   e. Prescription forgery

Section 5: Interventional procedures and neurostimulatory techniques for pain control; Complementary, nonpharmacologic treatments; Chronic pain and insomnia; Management of medication-related side effects

1. **In which TWO groups of patients is transcutaneous electrical nerve stimulation (TENS) contraindicated?**
   a. Patients with a pacemaker
   b. Age >65 years
   c. Age <14 years
   d. Pregnant women
   e. Alcoholics

2. **'Meralgia paresthetica' describes chronic pain from which nerve?**
   a. Lateral femoral cutaneous
   b. Greater occipital
   c. Ilioinguinal
   d. Genitofemoral
   e. Lesser occipital

3. **What is considered to be the most useful test for the diagnosis of discogenic pain?**
   a. MRI
   b. Physical examination, including the straight leg raising test
   c. X-ray
   d. Facet joint block
   e. Provocation discography

4. **Pain is associated with a range of distressing emotions, such as anxiety, depression, and fear of deterioration or death. Which of the following TWO questions should be asked to screen a patient for depression?**
   a. During the last month, how many times have you socialized with friends?
   b. During the last month, have you often been bothered by little interest or pleasure in doing things?
   c. During the last week, what was your alcohol intake?
   d. During the last month, have you often been bothered by feeling down, depressed, or hopeless?
   e. During the last week, have you often felt anxious or upset?

5. **Which of the following TWO statements regarding acupuncture are thought to be correct?**
   a. Randomized trials have shown acupuncture to be strongly effective in the treatment of diabetic neuropathy
   b. Acupuncture stimulates inhibitory Aβ and Aδ fibers entering the dorsal horn of the spinal cord
   c. Acupuncture is possibly efficacious in chronic low back pain
   d. Acupuncture is commonly associated with serious adverse effects, including infection and blood clots
   e. Acupuncture is an outmoded, unscientific technique, that has no place in contemporary pain treatment

6. **In fibromyalgia, sleep quality shows no correlation with symptom severity:**
   a. True
   b. False

7. **Medications used for chronic pain can either aid or hinder insomnia. Which of the following might be UNHELPFUL in a patient suffering from sleep difficulties, prompting a review of medication? The others can all aid sleep.**
   a. NSAIDs
   b. Anticonvulsants
   c. Opioids
   d. Antidepressants
   e. Dopaminergic drugs

8. **Many of the drug groups that are used in pain management have side effects, which can lead to complications. However, many of the adverse effects associated with pain medications can be prevented or minimized. Which TWO of the following are uncommon side effects of opioids? The rest are all found more often, and prophylaxis should be offered.**
   a. Constipation
   b. Nausea
   c. Urinary retention
   d. Dry mouth
   e. Pruritus

9. **Amitriptyline is the best proven antidepressant in neuropathic pain, but it has the most side effects (eg, dry mouth, drowsiness, postural hypotension). At which dose should amitriptyline be started?**
   a. 5–10 mg once daily
   b. 10–25 mg once daily
   c. 10–25 mg twice daily
   d. 25–50 mg twice daily
   e. 75 mg once daily

10. **In which patients is carbamazepine contraindicated? (Select all that apply.)**
    a. Bone marrow suppression
    b. Age >65 years
    c. Trigeminal neuralgia
    d. Known sensitivity to tricyclic compounds
    e. Liver abnormalities

Evaluation

At the conclusion of the activity, *Chronic Pain: A Primer for Physicians*, **go to:**
www.cecentral.com/getcredit/, enter the program code MEN07150,
and follow the online instructions to obtain credit.

Alternatively, complete the post-test answer sheet, program evaluation form, and registration form, and return to:
Attn: Distance Education
UKCPMCE [MEN07150]
One Quality Street, 6th Floor
Lexington, KY 40507-1428, USA
Fax: (859) 323-2920

Post-test answer sheet
Record your answers here by filling in the blank with the correct letter(s)
for the corresponding question:

Section 1: Physiology of pain; Epidemiology of chronic pain; Pain assessment
1. _____ 2. _____ 3. _____ 4. _____ 5. _____
6. _____ 7. _____ 8. _____ 9. _____ 10. _____

Section 2: Low back pain syndrome; Osteoarthritis; Ischemic pain syndromes; Visceral pain syndromes
1. _____ 2. _____ 3. _____ 4. _____ 5. _____
6. _____ 7. _____ 8. _____ 9. _____ 10. _____

Section 3: Neuropathic pain syndromes; Headache; Fibromyalgia; Cancer pain
1. _____ 2. _____ 3. _____ 4. _____ 5. _____
6. _____ 7. _____ 8. _____ 9. _____ 10. _____

Section 4: Breakthrough pain; Nonopioid analgesics and adjuvants; Opioids; Risk management with opioids
1. _____ 2. _____ 3. _____ 4. _____ 5. _____
6. _____ 7. _____ 8. _____ 9. _____ 10. _____
11. _____ 12. _____

Section 5: Interventional procedures and neurostimulatory techniques for pain control; Complementary, nonpharmacologic treatments; Chronic pain and insomnia; Management of medication-related side effects

1. _____ 2. _____ 3. _____ 4. _____ 5. _____
6. _____ 7. _____ 8. _____ 9. _____ 10. _____

Participants will receive a confidential report of their results, along with the correct answers to each question.

A certificate of credit will be sent to those who successfully complete the examination.

Program evaluation form

		Strongly agree				Strongly disagree
1.	The activity provided new information I had not yet acquired	1	2	3	4	5
2.	The activity helped to increase my knowledge and skills	1	2	3	4	5
3.	The activity content was educational and understandable	1	2	3	4	5
4.	The activity content met its objectives	1	2	3	4	5
5.	The amount of information presented was adequate for my needs	1	2	3	4	5
6.	I felt that I absorbed a reasonable amount of the presented materials	1	2	3	4	5
7.	The technical quality of the activity was acceptable	1	2	3	4	5
8.	I would recommend this program to my peers	1	2	3	4	5

9. Funding for this activity may have come from commercial sponsors. Do you think you were adequately informed of commercial sponsorship or faculty conflict of interest? Yes ☐ No ☐

10. Do you think that the overall activity was biased toward certain commercial products or services? Yes ☐ No ☐

Registration form

Name: ....

Affiliation: ....

Office address: ....

....

City: .... State: ....

Zip code: ....

Office phone: ....

Home phone: ....

Email: ....

Physician license no./State: ....

By signing this certificate, I attest that I have participated in the above continuing medical education program.

Signature: ....

Credit hours: ....